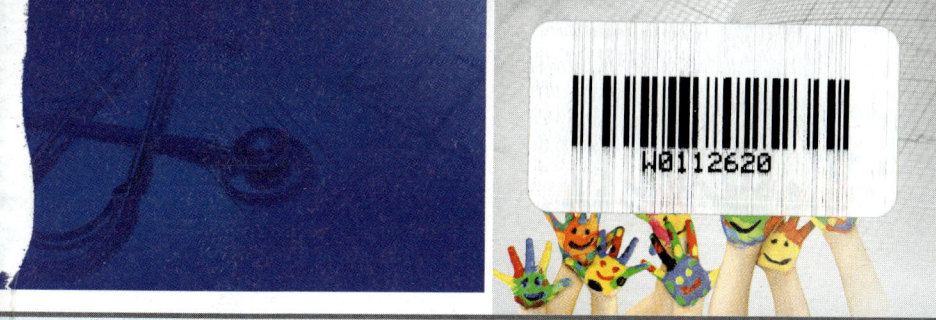

Paediatric
Electrocardiography

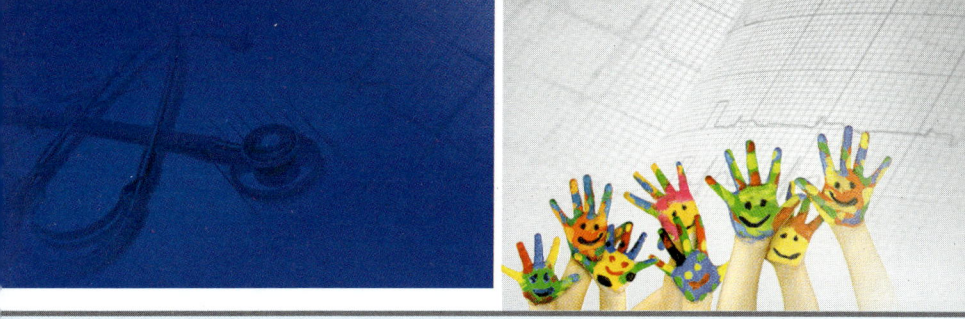

Paediatric
Electrocardiography

Sunil Natha Mhaske

MBBS MD (Paediatrics) MBA (Hospital Administration)
MA (Public Administration) PhD (Paediatrics)
Professor, Department of Paediatrics
Dean, Dr Vithalrao Vikhe Patil Foundation's Medical College
Ahmednagar, Maharashtra

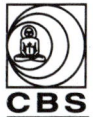

CBS

CBS Publishers & Distributors Pvt Ltd

New Delhi • Bengaluru • Chennai • Kochi • Kolkata • Mumbai
Hyderabad • Jharkhand • Nagpur • Patna • Pune • Uttarakhand

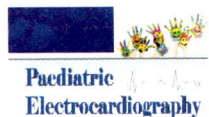

Paediatric Electrocardiography

ISBN: 978-93-89688-05-4

Copyright © Author and Publisher

First Edition: 2021

Published by Satish Kumar Jain and produced by Varun Jain for

CBS Publishers & Distributors Pvt Ltd

4819/XI Prahlad Street, 24 Ansari Road, Daryaganj, New Delhi 110 002, India
Ph: 011-23289259, 23266861, 23266867   Website: www.cbspd.com
Fax: 011-23243014   e-mail: delhi@cbspd.com; cbspubs@airtelmail.in
Corporate Office: 204 FIE, Industrial Area, Patparganj, Delhi 110 092

Ph: 011-4934 4934   Fax: 011-4934 4935   e-mail: publishing@cbspd.com; publicity@cbspd.com

Branches

- **Bengaluru:** Seema House 2975, 17th Cross, K.R. Road,
  Banasankari 2nd Stage, Bengaluru 560 070, Karnataka
  Ph: +91-80-26771678/79   Fax: +91-80-26771680   e-mail: bangalore@cbspd.com
- **Chennai:** 7, Subbaraya Street, Shenoy Nagar, Chennai 600 030, Tamil Nadu
  Ph: +91-44-26680620, 26681266   Fax: +91-44-42032115   e-mail: chennai@cbspd.com
- **Kochi:** 42/1325, 1326, Power House Road, Opp KSEB, Kochi 682 018, Kerala, India
  Ph: +91-484-4059061-65   Fax: +91-484-4059065   e-mail: kochi@cbspd.com
- **Kolkata:** 6/B, Ground Floor, Rameswar Shaw Road, Kolkata 700 014, West Bengal
  Ph: +91-33-22891126, 22891127, 22891128   e-mail: kolkata@cbspd.com
- **Mumbai:** 83-C, Dr E Moses Road, Worli, Mumbai 400018, Maharashtra
  Ph: +91-22-24902340/41   Fax: +91-22-24902342   e-mail: mumbai@cbspd.com

Representatives

| • Hyderabad | 0-9885175004 | • Jharkhand | 0-9811541605 | • Nagpur | 0-9421945513 |
| • Patna | 0-9334159340 | • Pune | 0-9623451994 | • Uttarakhand | 0-9716462459 |

Printed At : Goyal Offset Works (P) Limited

to

---

all my postgraduate students
Department of Paediatrics, Dr Vithalrao Vikhe Patil
Foundation's Medical College and Hospital
Ahmednagar, Maharashtra, India

Preface

Electrocardiograph is very important and old diagnostic tool in medical field. It has played an important role in the understanding of cardiovascular diseases. In paediatric field electrocardiograph has been time-tested investigation. Electrocardiography is a quick, simple, painless procedure in which the heart's electrical impulses are amplified and recorded.

There was need of such book for undergraduate and postgraduate students as well as paediatric practitioners. In view of it, I have made attempt by writing this book *Paediatric Electrocardiography*.

I am very thankful to Dr Sujay Vikhe Patil (CEO, Dr Vithalrao Vikhe Patil Foundation, Ahmednagar), Dr B Sadananda (Secretary General, Dr Vithalrao Vikhe Patil Foundation, Ahmednagar), Dr Abhijit Diwate (Deputy Director, Dr Vithalrao Vikhe Patil Foundation, Ahmednagar).

In the process of writing I had been very much supported by my postgraduate students: Dr Liza Bulsara, Dr Ninza Rawal, Dr Bipin Rathod, Dr Prajakta Ghatge, Dr Amit Italia and Dr Vinit Gupta. I am also thankful to Dr Rucha Tipare and Dr Kajal Jain.

I am heartfully thankful to my wife Dr Rekha and children Prabhat and Rucha.

Any suggestions or comments are welcomed in the process of upgradation of book on mail id sunilmhaske1970@gmail.com.

Sunil Natha Mhaske

Contents

Abbreviations

LVH: Left ventricular hypertrophy

RVH: Right ventricular hypertrophy

LBBB: Left bundle branch block

RBBB: Right bundle branch block

WPW: Wolff-Parkinson-White syndrome

QTc: Corrected QT interval

PVC: Premature ventricular contraction

AV: Atrioventricular

bpm: Beats per minute

msec or ms: Milliseconds

sec: Second or seconds

TOF: Tetralogy of Fallot

RPL: Right precordial leads

LPL: Left precordial leads

SVT: Supraventricular tachycardia

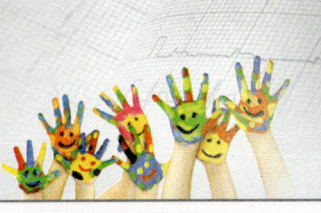

1

Introduction to Electrocardiography

Pioneers of Electrocardiography

1791: Galvani (Italy)—first showed electromotor activity in the leg muscle of the frog.

1820: Hans Christian Orsted (Danish physicist)—discovered the phenomenon of electromagnetism.

1840: Carlo Matteucci—demonstrated that every beat of a frog's heart generates electricity which was the first steps towards electrocardiography.

1957: Norman Holter—invented the dynamic ECG (Holter ECG) portable device for continuous monitoring of various electrical activities of the cardiovascular system for 24 hours.

1872: Gabriel Lippmann (French physicist) invented the capillary electrometer.

1876: Etienne-Jules Marey (French physiologist)—used the Lippmann electrometer to record electrical activity in an exposed heart of a frog. It was the true beginning of modern electrocardiography.

1882: John Burdon-Sanderson—while working with frogs he coined the term isoelectric interval.

1899: Karel Frederik Wenckebach (Dutch scholar)—he worked on irregular pulse and impairment of atrioventricular conduction which leads to progressive lengthening and blockage of atrioventricular conduction in frogs (Wenckebach block: Mobitz type I).

1888–1979: Bernard A Robinson—to the early development of the electrocardiograph.

Alexander Muirhead

- Born on 26th May 1848 in Scotland.
- Electrical engineer by profession.
- He invented the first human electrocardiogram.
- He died on 13th December 1920 in Short lands, Kent.

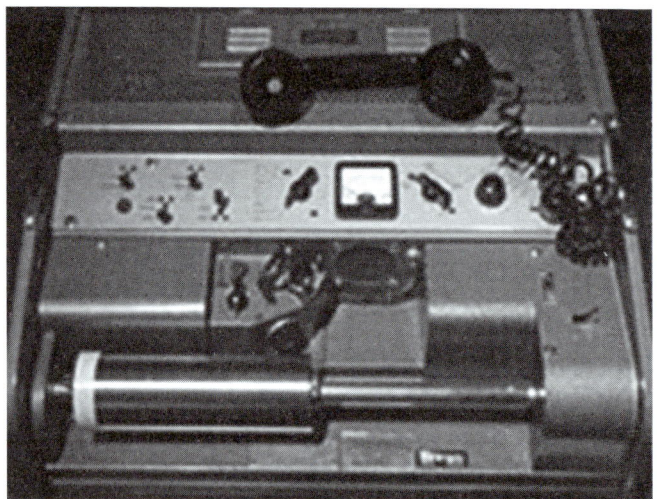

Fig. 1.1: Muirhead fax machine

Augustus Desire Waller

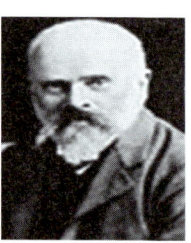

- Born on 18 July 1856
- He was a British physiologist.
- In 1887, he used a capillary electrometer to record the first human electrocardiogram.
- He created the first practical ECG machine with surface electrodes.
- He died on 11 March 1922.

Willem Einthoven

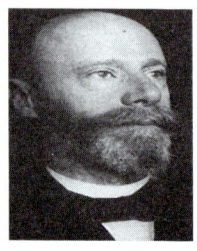

- Born on 21 May 1860
- In 1903, he invented the first practical electrocardiogram.
- He assigned letters P, Q, R, S and T to various deflections.

- Einthoven's triangle—imaginary inverted equilateral triangle centered on the chest and the points being the standard leads on the arms and leg.
- He described the electrocardiographic features of a number of cardiovascular disorders.
- In 1924, he was awarded with the Nobel Prize in Medicine for inventing the first practical system of electrocardiography used in medical diagnosis.
- He died on 29 September 1927.

Taro Takemi

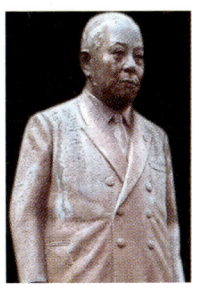

- Born on 7th August 1904.
- In 1937, he built the first portable electrocardiograph.
- He was honored with Italian Order of Merit and Silver Medal from Pope Paul VI.
- Died on 29th December 1983.

Introduction to Electrocardiogram

- Electrocardiography is a Greek word.
- Electro—electrical activity, kardio—heart, graph—to write.
- It is a sophisticated galvanometer, a sensitive electromagnet.
- A process of recording the electrical activity of the heart is known as electrocardiogram (ECG or EKG).
- Electrodes detect the electrical changes on the skin that arise from the heart muscle's depolarization during heartbeat.
- Goal of ECG—to obtain information of structure and function of the heart.
- Continuous ECG monitoring
  - To monitor critically ill patients
  - General anesthesia
  - Cardiac dysrhythmia
- Clinical cardiac electrophysiology
  - To measure the electrical activity
  - Catheter is inserted through the femoral vein
  - Electrodes record the direction of electrical activity of heart.

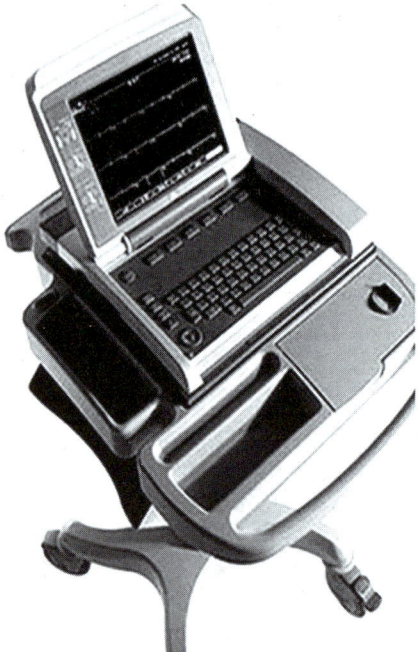

Fig. 1.2: ECG machine

- ECG voltages measures hundreds of microvolts up to 1 milli-volt (the small square on a standard ECG is 100 microvolts).

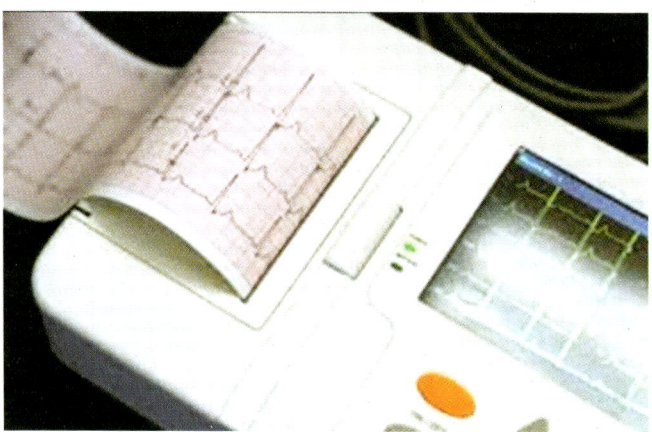

Fig. 1.3: ECG machine

Electrophysiology of ECG

- Cardiac stimulus is generated in the sinoatrial (SA) node.
- SA node is located in right atrium.
- Stimulus then spread through right atrium to left atrium
- Then it spreads through atrioventricular node and the bundle of His (AV junction).

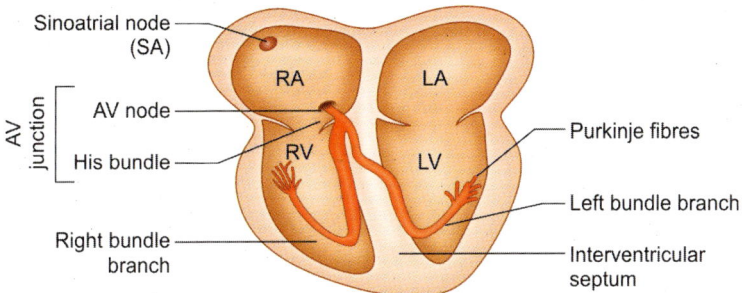

Fig. 1.4: Cardiac chambers

- Stimulus then passes through left and right ventricle by the way of left and right bundle branches (bundle of His).
- Finally cardiac stimulus spreads through the ventricular muscle cells through Purkinje fibres.

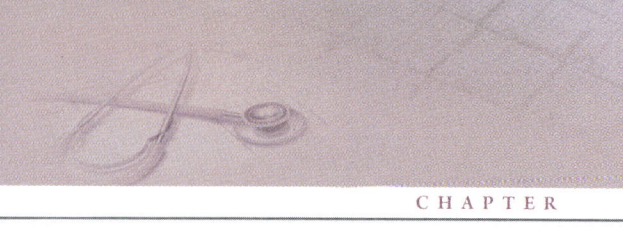
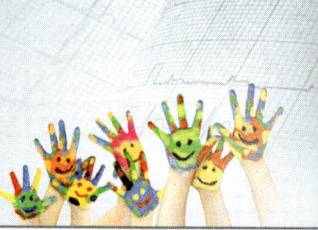

Electrodes and Leads

Electrodes

- A conductive pad in contact with the body that makes an electrical circuit with the electrocardiograph.
- On a standard 12-lead EKG there are 10 electrodes.

Leads: Einthoven's Triangle

- Source of measurement of a vector
- Limb leads: Bipolar → comparison between two electrodes
- Precordial leads → unipolar → compared to a common lead
- Three sets: Limb, augmented limb and precordial

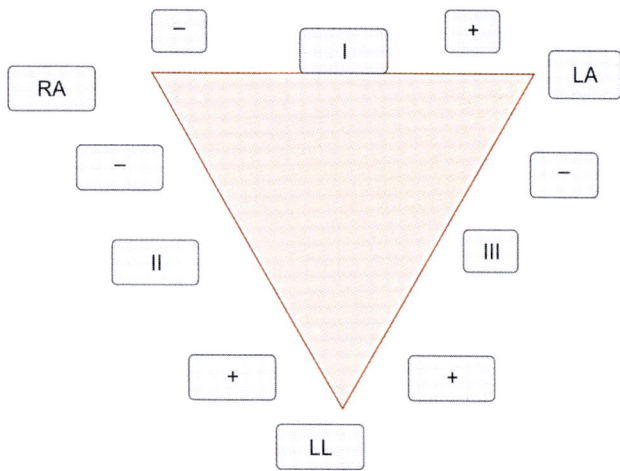

Fig. 2.1: Leads: Einthoven's triangle

- In 12-lead ECG →
  - Three limb leads
  - Three augmented limb leads arranged like spokes of a wheel in the coronal plane—vertical
  - Six precordial leads that lie on the perpendicular transverse plane—horizontal.

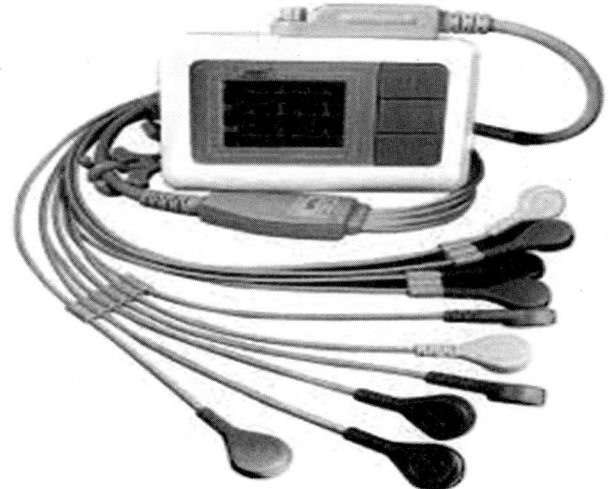

Fig. 2.2: ECG machine with leads

- Limb electrodes can be placed
  - Far down on the limbs or
  - Close to the hips/shoulders placed symmetrically.

12 leads in a 12-lead ECG

Electrode	Placement
RA	Right arm
LA	Left arm
RL	Right leg-lateral calf muscle
LL	Left leg
V1	Fourth intercostals space—right of the sternum
V2	Fourth intercostal space—left of the sternum
V3	Between leads V2 and V4

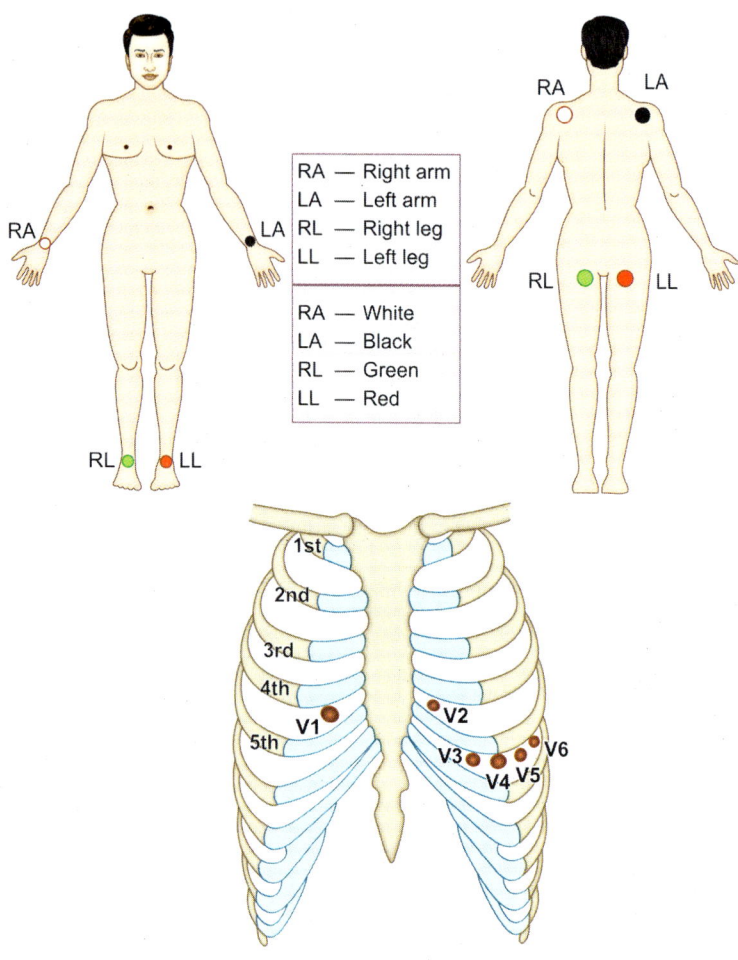

Fig. 2.3: Lead positions

V4	Fifth intercostal space in the mid-clavicular line.
V5	Horizontally even with V4, in the left anterior axillary line.
V6	Horizontally even with V4 and V5 in the midaxillary line.

1. *Limb Leads*

- Leads I, II and III
- One on each arm and one on the left leg.
- Limb leads form the Einthoven's triangle.

- Lead I is the voltage between the (positive) left arm (LA) electrode and right arm (RA) electrode.
- Lead II is the voltage between the (positive) left leg (LL) electrode and the right arm (RA) electrode.
- Lead III is the voltage between the (positive) left leg (LL) electrode and the left arm (LA) electrode.

2. Augmented Limb Leads

A. Lead augmented vector right (aVR)
  - Positive electrode on the right arm
  - Negative pole is a combination of the left arm electrode and the left leg electrode
B. Lead augmented vector left (aVL)
  - Positive electrode on the left arm
  - Negative pole is a combination of the right arm electrode and the left leg electrode.
C. Augmented vector foot (aVF)
  - Positive electrode on the left leg
  - Negative pole is a combination of the right arm electrode and the left arm electrode.

3. Precordial Leads

- Lie in the transverse (horizontal) plane
- Perpendicular to the other six leads
- Act as the positive poles.

4. Specialized Leads

- V5R-dextrocardia
- V7 to V9-posterior myocardial infarction
- Lewis lead-study pathological rhythms arising in the right atrium.
- Esophageal lead-inserted to a part of the esophagus for cardiac arrhythmias, atrial flutter, AV nodal tachycardia , Wolff-Parkinson-White syndrome, supraventricular tachycardia.

Lead Locations on Standard 12-lead ECG Report

- 2.5 second tracing of each of the twelve leads

- Tracings are arranged in a grid of four columns and three rows
- First column—limb leads (I, II, and III)
- Second column—augmented limb leads (aVR, aVL, and aVF)
- Last two columns—precordial leads (V1–V6)
- Fourth or fifth row—rhythm strip.

Sequence of Tracing

I	aVR	V1	V4
II	aVL	V2	V5
III	aVF	V3	V6

Electrical Activity of Leads

- Leads II, III and aVF—diaphragmatic surface of heart
- I, aVL, V5 and V6—lateral wall of left ventricle
- V1 and V2—interventricular septum
- V3 and V4—Sternocostal surface of heart.

15-lead ECG

- Sensitivity of a single 12-lead ECG for the diagnosis of acute MI is relatively weak.
- Standard 12-lead ECG does not include posterior leads so the changes associated with necrosis in this region are reflected in the anterior leads.
- Use of the 15-lead ECG confirms the posterior MI and is superior to the findings in the anterior leads.
- The use of the 15-lead ECG contributes to a faster and more accurate diagnosis of STEMI facilitating the prompt reperfusion therapy.
- Routine use of 15-lead ECG for ICCU department patients with chest pain should be recommended.

Electromagnetism of Heart

- Heart is the most powerful generator of electromagnetic energy in the human body.
- It produces the largest rhythmic electromagnetic field of any of the body's organs.

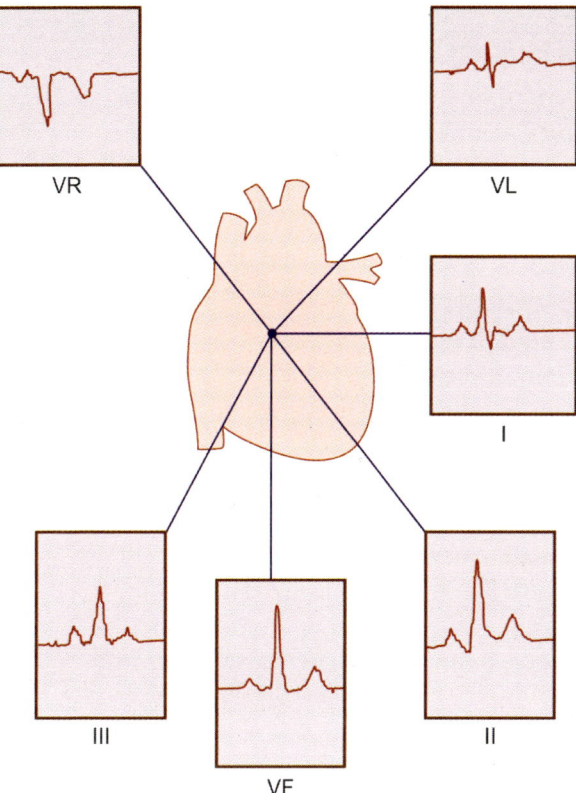

Fig. 2.4: Electromagnetism of heart

- Heart's electrical field is about 60 times greater in amplitude that the electrical activity generated by the brain.
- This is measured in the form of an electrocardiogram.
- It can be detected in all directions by using SQUID-based.
- Depolarization of the heart toward the positive electrode → positive deflection.
- Depolarization of the heart away from the positive electrode → negative deflection.
- Repolarization of the heart toward the positive electrode → negative deflection.
- Repolarization of the heart away from the positive electrode → positive deflection.

Normal Rhythm Produces

- P wave—atrial depolarization
- QRS complex—ventricular depolarization.
- T wave—ventricular repolarization.
- U wave—papillary muscle repolarization.

ECG Paper

- Divided as small and large squares.
- Small square is 1 mm square.
- Large square is 5 mm square.
- Horizontal measurement—time
- Vertical measurement—amplitude
- Paper speed is 25 mm/sec
- That means five large squares represent 1 second.
- One large square represents 0.20 sec or 200 ms.
- One small square represents 0.04 sec or 40 ms.
- Small box: 1 mm × 1 mm in size and of 0.1 mV × 0.04 seconds width
- Large box: 5 mm × 5 mm in size and of 0.5 mV × 0.2 seconds width.

ECG on Graph Paper at Standard Scale

- Each 1 mm (one small box on the standard ECG paper) represents 40 milliseconds of time on the x-axis, and
- 0.1 millivolts on the y-axis.

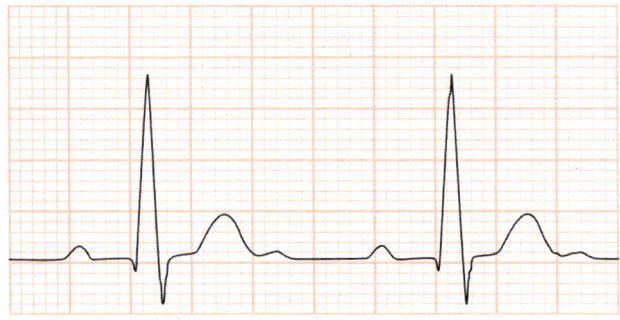

Fig. 2.5: ECG on graph paper at standard scale

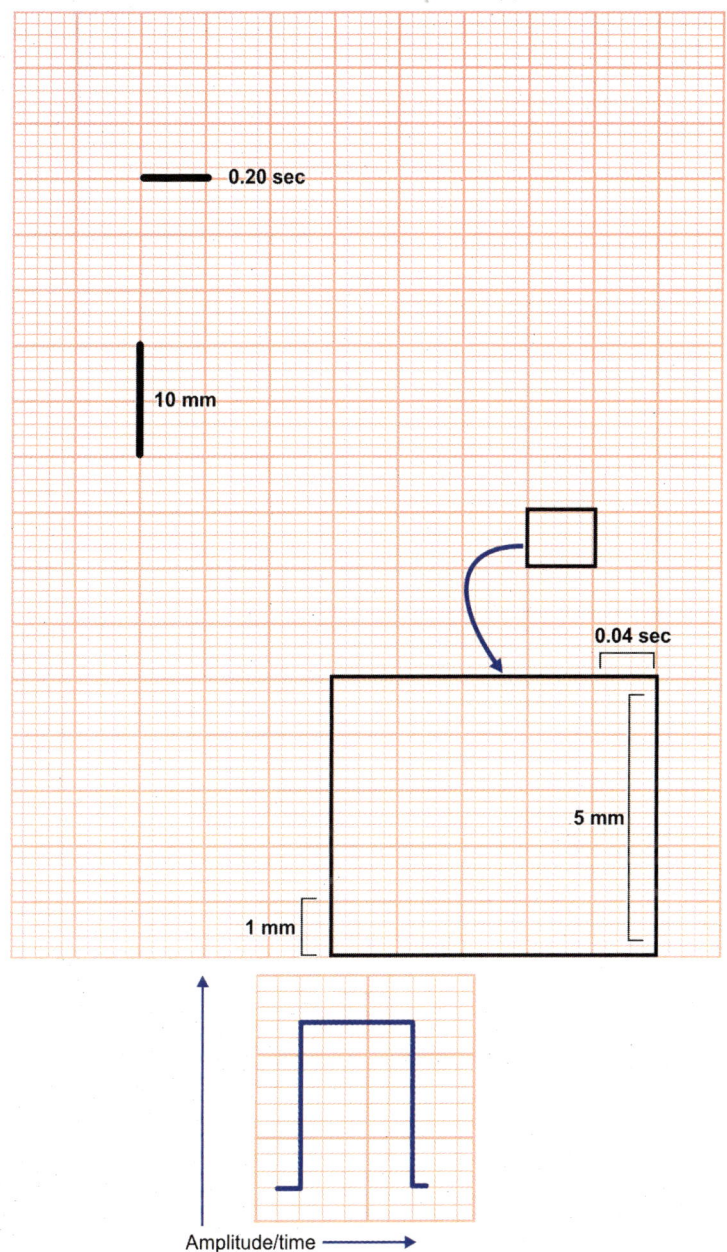

Fig. 2.6: ECG on graph paper

Artifacts

- Are distorted signals caused by a muscle movement or interference from an electrical device.
- ECG tracing is affected by patient motion.
- Shivering or tremors can create the illusion of cardiac dysrhythmia.
- Improper lead placement also creates artifacts.

Gel

- Contains potassium chloride/silver chloride
- Permits electron conduction from the skin to the wire and to the electrocardiogram.

Interpretation of ECG

- Check the name on the top of the ECG
- Check the date—is this the one you ordered?
- Check for old ECGs—just like a chest X-ray, it is always a good idea to compare with an old one.
- Check for the age of the patient—the heart physiology and the normal values differ in different age groups in the paediatrics.

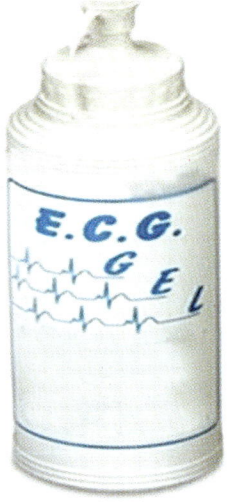

Fig. 2.7: ECG gel

Heart rate	Rhythm	PR interval
P wave size	QRS width (interval)	QT/QTc interval
QRS voltage	Mean QRS voltage electrical axis	R wave progression in chest leads
Abnormal Q waves	ST segments	T waves
U waves		

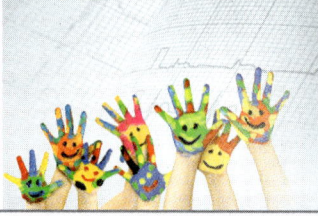

Axis of Heart

- Heart has several axes.
- Common is the axis of the QRS complex.
- Axis means a degree of deviation from zero.
- QRS axis → direction of the ventricular depolarization in frontal plane.

Ventricular (QRS) Axis

- Is determined by looking at the QRS complex
- Represents ventricular depolarization

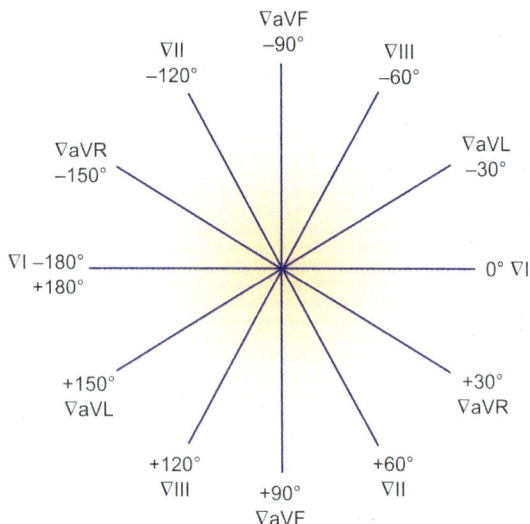

Fig. 3.1: Axes of heart

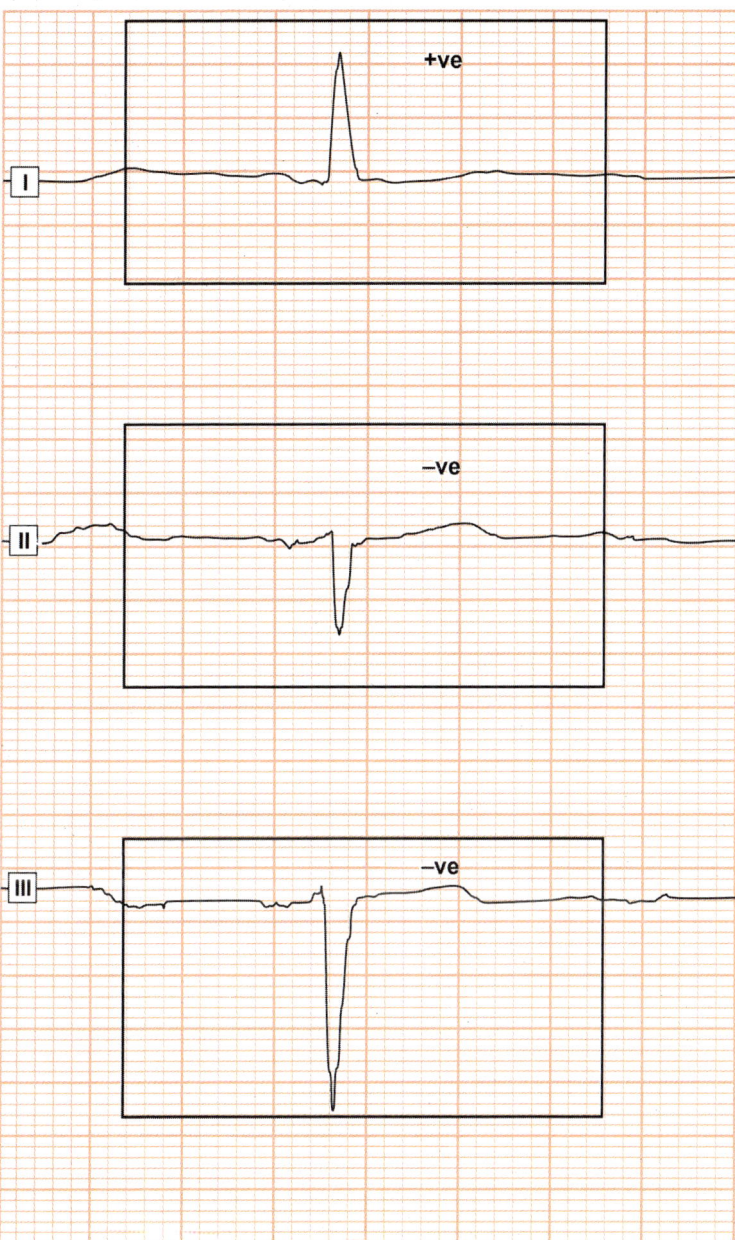

Fig. 3.2: Left axis deviation

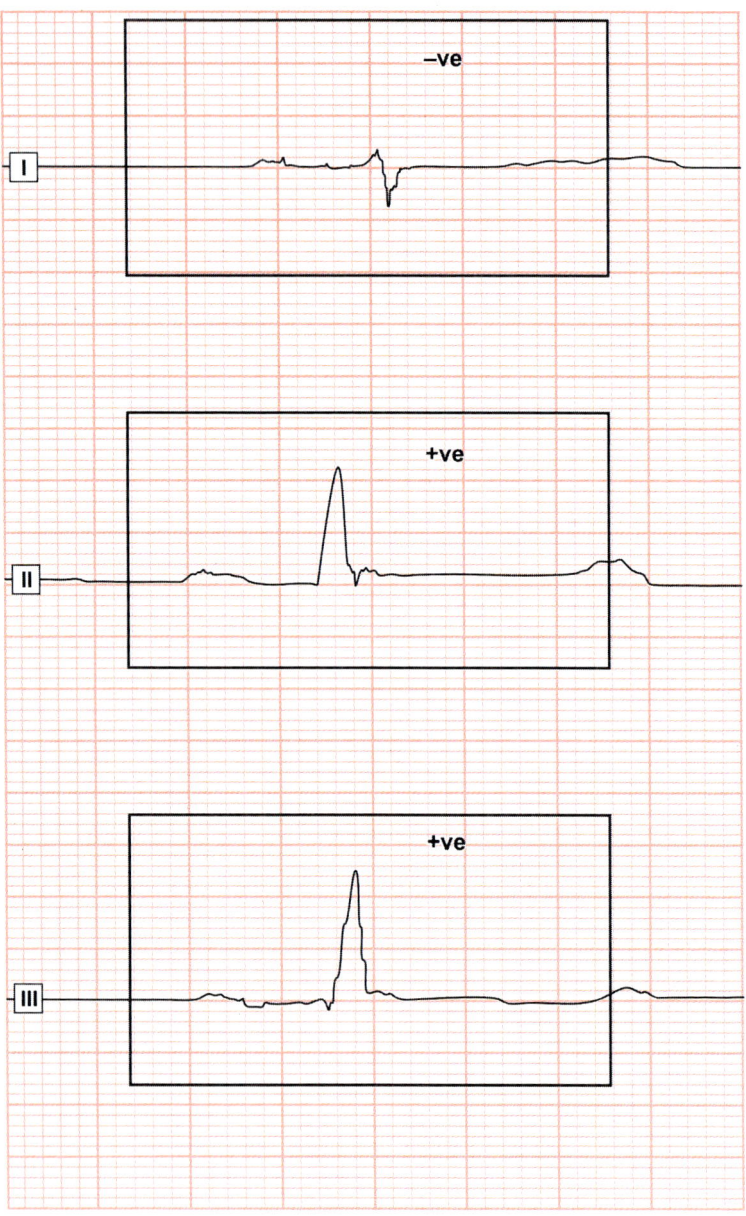

Fig. 3.3: Right axis deviation

- Also referred to as the QRS axis.
- It signifies the sum of all individual vectors generated by the depolarization waves of ventricular myocytes.
- It is determined indirectly by evaluating the vectors produced under the electrodes.
- Positive QRS complex in a lead has a ventricular axis that is in the same direction to that lead.
- Negative QRS complex in a lead has a ventricular axis that is in the opposite direction to that lead.
- QRS complex is isoelectric in a lead—ventricular axis is perpendicular (90°) to that lead.

Types

1. Normal QRS axis: –30° to 105° with 0° being along lead I (positive in lead I and lead II), generally down and to the left.
2. Right axis deviation: Beyond +105° to +180°
3. Left axis deviation: Beyond –30° to –90° (QRS complex positive in lead I and negative in leads aVF and II)
4. Indeterminate axis/north–west axis/extreme axis deviation: +180° to –90°.

Left axis deviation	Right axis deviation
Lt. ventricular hypertrophy	Rt. ventricular hypertrophy
Lt. anterior fascicular block	Lt. posterior fascicular block
Old inferior myocardial infarction	Old lateral myocardial infarction
Wolff-Parkinson-White syndrome	COPD
Ostium primumatrial septal defect	Pulmonary arterial hypertension
Normal in obesity	Large pulmonary embolism
Emphysema	Left-sided myocardial infarction
	Left posterior fascicular block
Indeterminate axis—rare	Tall and thin persons
	Situs inversus

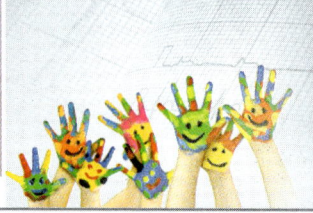

4

Cardiac Rate and Rhythm

Rate

- Normally heart rate is the rate in which the sinoatrial node depolarizes.
- Usual paper speed is 25 mm/sec
- 1 mm (small square) = 0.04 sec
- 5 mm (big square) = 0.2 sec
- Regular rhythms: 300/number of large squares in between each consecutive R wave.
- Resting heart rate varies with age:

Newborn	110–150 bpm
2 years	85–125 bpm
4 years	75–115 bpm
6 years+	60–100 bpm

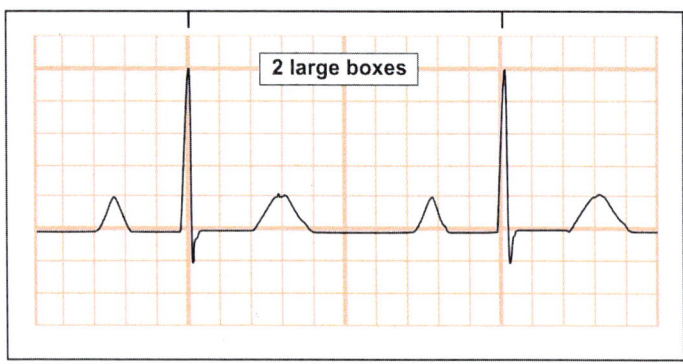

Fig. 4.1: Cardiac rate

Rhythm

- Physiologic rhythm of the heart is known as normal sinus rhythm
- Normal sinus rhythm produces the prototypical pattern of P wave, QRS complex, and T wave.
- **Normal sinus rhythm**
  - Atrial depolarization starts from the sinoatrial node
  - P wave preceding each QRS complex, with a constant PR interval
  - Normal P wave axis (0 to + 90°)
  - P wave is upright in leads I and aVF.
  - P waves and QRS complexes appear one-to-one.

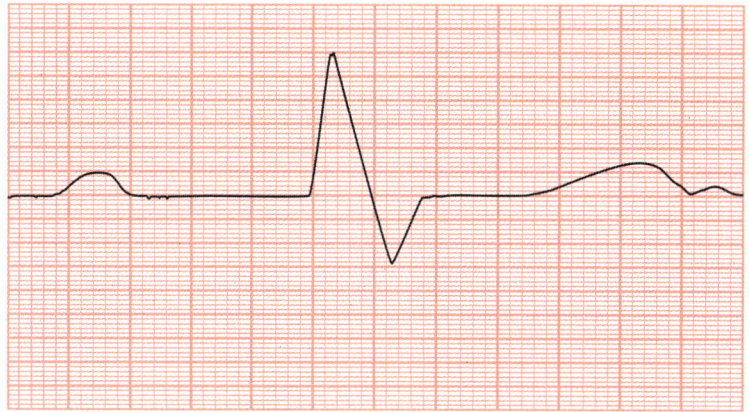

Fig. 4.2: Normal sinus rhythm

- **Sinus arrhythmias**
  - Alternating periods of slow and rapid rates.
  - Due to irregular fluctuating discharge of the sinoatrial node.
  - Associated with phases of respiration
  - Faster rate—inspiration and slower rate-expiration
  - Absent P waves with 'irregularly irregular' QRS complexes—atrial fibrillation
  - Saw tooth pattern with QRS complexes—atrial flutter
  - Sine wave pattern—ventricular flutter

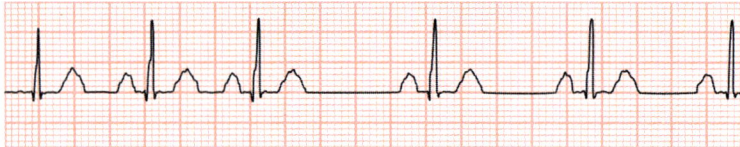

Fig. 4.3: Sinus arrhythmias

- Absent P waves with wide QRS complexes with fast rate-ventricular tachycardia.
- **Sinus tachycardia**
  - SA node discharges at faster than 100/min in adults
  - Normal P-QRS-T complex in rapid succession
  - Seen in emotions, respiration, exercise, thyrotoxicosis, toxemia, cardiac failure.

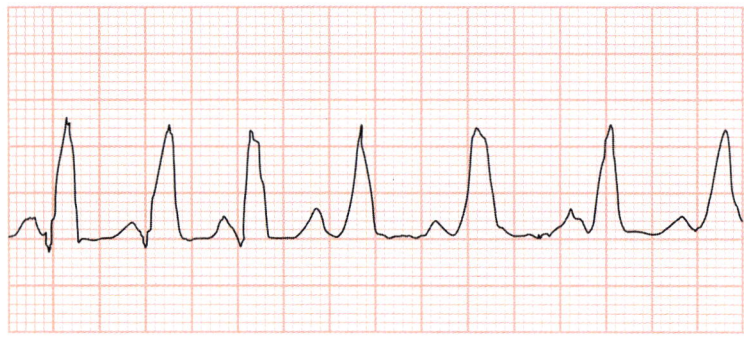

Fig. 4.4: Sinus tachycardia

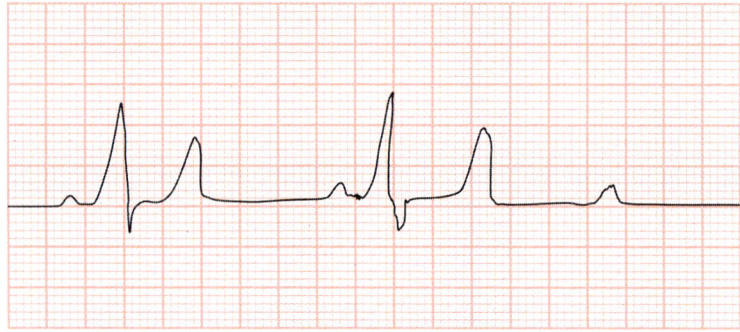

Fig. 4.5: Sinus bradycardia

- **Sinus bradycardia**
  - SA node discharges at a slower than 60/min
  - Normal P-QRS-T complex in slow succession
  - Seen in myxedema, obstructive jaundice, uremia, increased intracranial pressure, glaucoma.

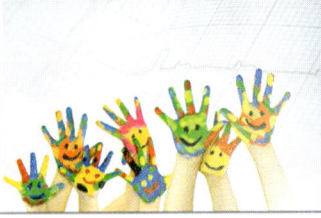

5

Waves of Electrocardiogram

- ECG cycles consist of five waves: P, Q, R, S, T corresponding to different phases of the heart activities.
- P wave represents the normal atrium (upper heart chambers) depolarization.
- QRS complex (one single heartbeat) corresponds to the depolarization of the right and left ventricles.
- T wave represents the re-polarization of the ventricles.

Wave	Amplitude
P wave	0.25 mV
R wave	1.6 mV
Q wave	25% of R wave
T wave	0.1 to 0.5 mV

Interval	Duration
PR wave	0.12–0.2 sec
QT wave	0.35–0.44 sec
ST wave	0.05–0.15 sec
P wave interval	0.11 sec

P Wave

- Represents atrial depolarization which results in atrial contraction.
- Normally right atrium depolarizes slightly earlier than left atrium
- Depolarization wave originated in the sinoatrial node and spreads to right atrium and then to left atrium.

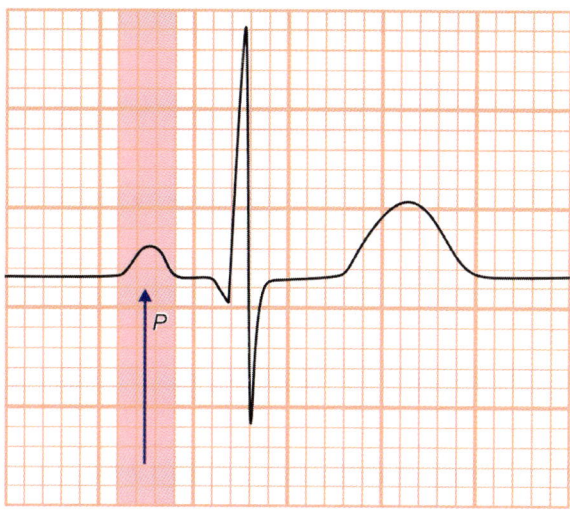

Fig. 5.1: Waves of electrocardiogram

- Depolarization is carried through atria along semi-specialized conduction pathways (Bachmann's bundle) which results in uniform shaped waves.
- Lewis lead: If P waves are not clearly delineated in the surface ECG, this lead is used for better visualization of P waves.

P wave	Condition
Peaked P waves (>2.5 mm)	Right atrial enlargement (*P pulmonale*)
Increased amplitude of P wave	Hypokalemia—right atrial enlargement
Decreased amplitude of P wave	Hyperkalemia
Bifid P waves (*P mitrale*)	Left-atrial abnormality—dilatation/hypertrophy
Multiple ectopic foci → 3 different shaped P waves	Multifocal atrial tachycardia—chronic obstructive lung disease
Saw-tooth shaped baseline	Flutter waves of atrial flutter
Absence of the P wave with flat baseline	Fine atrial fibrillation, sinoatrial arrest
Variable morphologies of P waves	Wandering pacemaker, multifocal atrial tachycardia

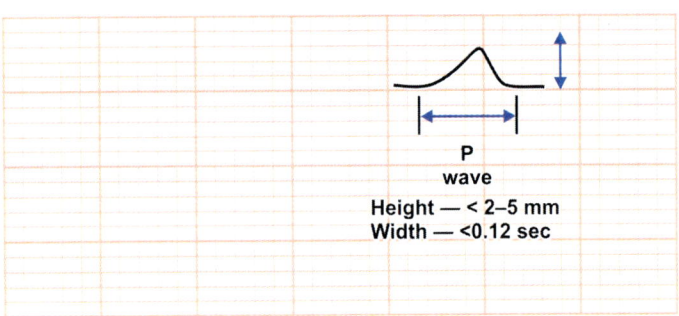

Fig. 5.2: P wave

P Wave Axis

Normal	+40° to 60° clockwise
P pulmonale—acquired right heart disease	+60° to +90°
P wave emphysema	0° to +90°
P congenital—congenital heart disease	+40° to +70° clockwise
Left atrial enlargement	+45° to –30° counterclockwise
Mirror image dextrocardia, reversed arm electrodes	+120° clockwise to +150°

Ta Wave

- It indicates atrial repolarization.
- Occurs with a mean of 320 ms after the end of the P wave.
- Duration of 2–3 times that of the P wave.
- Polarityis opposite to that of the P wave.
- It is represented on the surface ECG by a so-called.
- It is a normal phenomenon
- Nadir of the Ta wave can occur just after the QRS complex.
- It causes ST depression similar toand mistaken as cardiac ischemia.

PR Interval

- It is measured in milliseconds.
- From the beginning of the P wave till the beginning of the QRS complex.

- That is onset of atrial depolarization till the beginning of onset of ventricular depolarization
- Normal duration—120 to 200 ms.

Long PR interval (>200 ms)	First degree heart block, hypokalemia, acute rheumatic fever, carditis with Lyme disease
Short PR interval (<120 ms)	Wolff-Parkinson-White syndrome, Lown-Ganong-Levine syndrome, junctional rhythms
Variable PR interval	Heart block
Depressed PR segment	Atrial injury, pericarditis

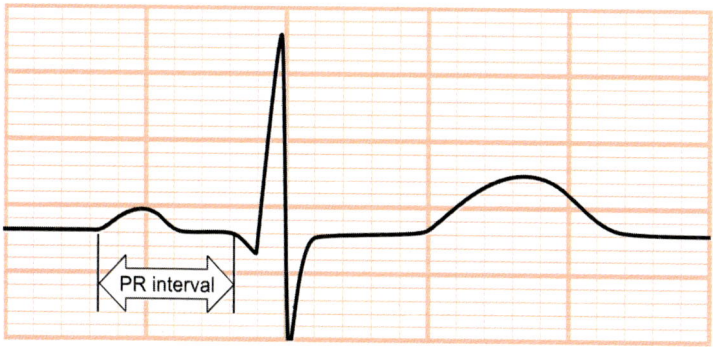

Fig. 5.3: PR interval

QRS Complex

- It corresponds to the depolarization of the right and left ventricles of heart.
- Depolarization of the heart ventricles occurs almost simultaneously via the Bundle of His and Purkinje fibers.
- Ventricles have more muscle mass than the atria → QRS complex is larger than the P wave.
- Q, R, and S waves occur in rapid succession.
- It reflects as a single event.
- Normal duration—80 to 120 ms (0.06–0.10 sec)

Short duration	Children, physical activity
Prolonged duration	Hyperkalemia or bundle branch block
Increased QRS amplitude	Cardiac hypertrophy

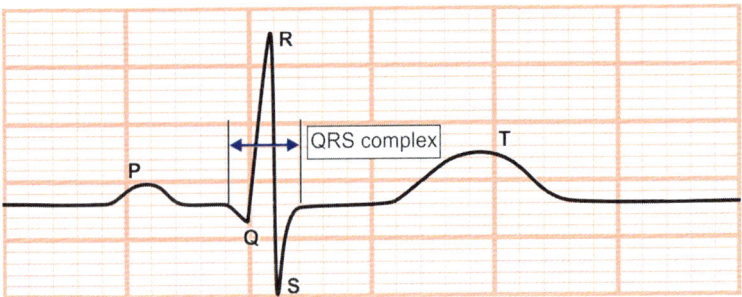

Fig. 5.4: QRS complex

- Q wave is a downward deflection after the P wave.
- R wave is a upward deflection after Q wave.
- S wave is a downward deflection after the R wave.
- T wave follows the S wave.
- U wave occurs in some cases as a additional wave that follows the T wave.
- RSR' pattern—abnormal second upward deflection within the QRS complex (R')—bundle branch block
- Not every QRS complex contains a Q wave, an R wave, and an S wave.
- Monomorphic—all QRS waves in a single lead being similar in shape.
- Polymorphic—QRS change from complex to complex.
- Algorithm for QRS complex detection—Pan-Tompkins.

Q Wave

- It is the downward deflection after the P wave.
- It occurs during interventricular septum depolarization (septal Q wave).
- It is seen in lateral leads I, aVL, V5 and V6.
- Pathologic Q wave: > 0.04 s (40 ms) in width and >2 mm in amplitude → markers of previous myocardial infarctions (ST elevation).

R Wave

Poor R wave progression
- R wave is less than 2–4 mm in leads V3 or V4.

- Rs complex would be positively deflected.
- rS complex would be negatively deflected.
- Presence of a reversed R wave progression.

Faulty ECG recording	Anterior myocardial infarction
Left bundle branch block	Wolff-Parkinson-White syndrome
Right and left ventricular hypertrophy	

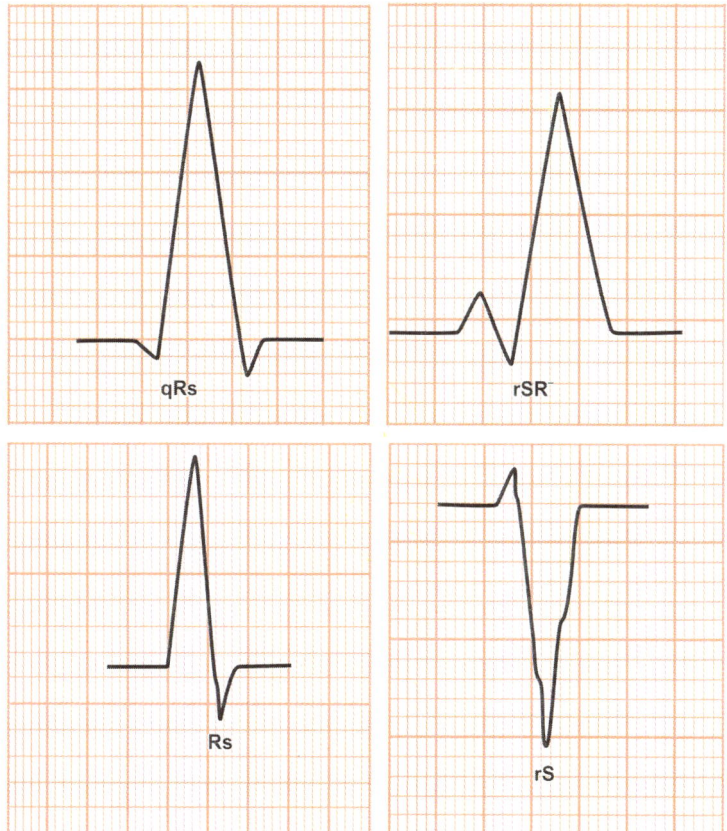

Fig. 5.5: R wave types

J-point

- It is the point where the QRS complex meets the ST seg-ment.

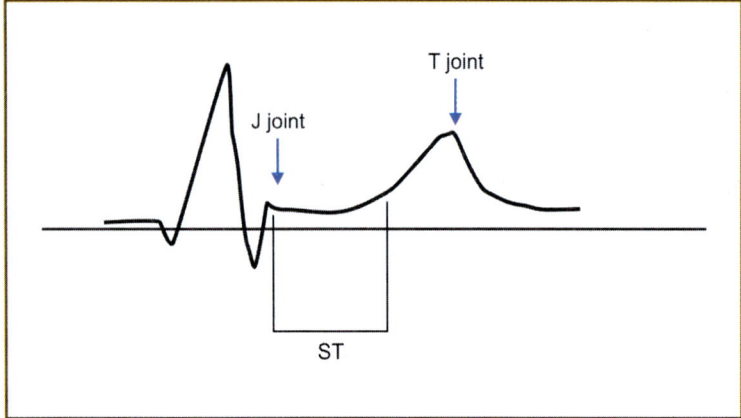

Fig. 5.6: J point

- ST segment is horizontal and forms a sharp angle with the last part of the QRS complex.
- First point of inflection of the upstroke of the S wave.
- Point at which the ECG trace becomes more horizontal than vertical.

JT Interval
- Useful when the QT interval is prolonged secondary to a prolonged QRS complex.
- Measured from the J point (junction between S wave and ST segment) to the end of T wave.
- Normal JTc (mean +/–SD): 0.32 +/– 0.02 seconds.
- Prolonged JTc has the same significance as the prolonged QTc interval.

ST Segment
- It represents the depolarization of ventricles.
- ST segment connects QRS complex and T wave.
- Duration—0.080 to 0.120 sec (80 to 120 ms)
- Starts at the J point and ends at the beginning of the T wave.
- Normally have slight upward concavity.

Flat, downsloping or depressed ST segments	Coronary ischemia
Elevated ST-elevation	Transmural myocardial infarction
ST depression	Subendocardial myocardial infarction, hypokalemia, digitalis toxicity

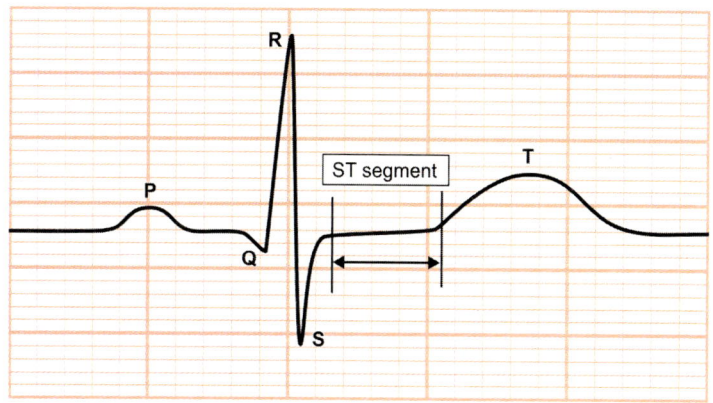

Fig. 5.7: ST segment

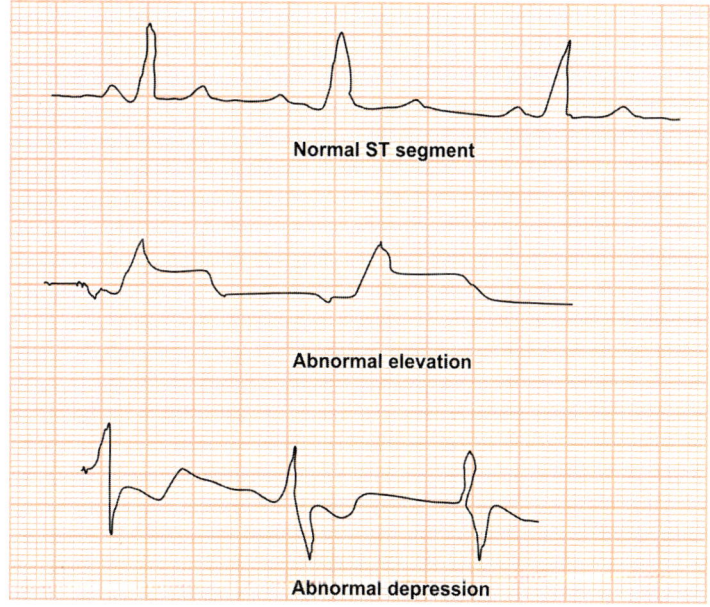

Fig. 5.8: ST segment abnormalities

T wave

- T wave—follows the S wave.
- It represents repolarization of ventricles.
- Positive T wave—in most of the leads.
- Negative T wave—lead aVR
- Positive, negative or biphasic T wave—lead V1
- T-wave inversion /negative T waves—coronary ischemia, Wellens' syndrome, left ventricular hypertrophy, CNS disorder.
- Tall and narrow symmetrical T waves—hyperkalemia.
- Flat T waves—coronary ischemia or hypokalemia.
- Hyperacute T wave—broad base and slight asymmetry-acute myocardial infarction, Prinzmetal angina.
- Appropriate T wave discordance—T wave is deflected opposite the terminal deflection of the QRS complex, e.g. bundle branch block.

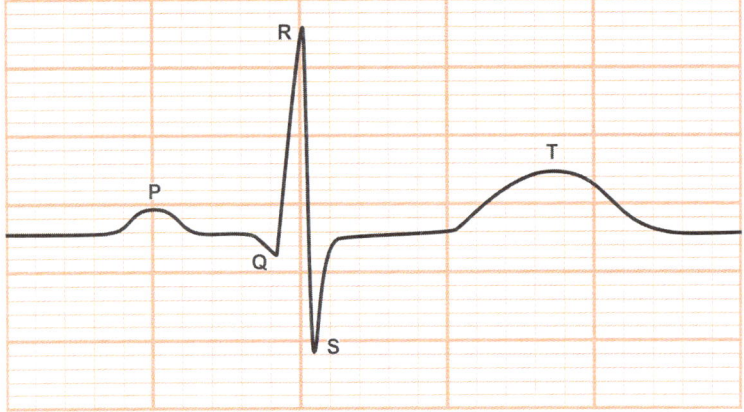

Fig. 5.9: T wave

QT Interval

- It is the measure of the time between the start of the Q wave and the end of the T wave.
- It represents ventricular depolarization and repolarization
- Commonly measured in lead II, I and V5.
- Faster the heart rate the shorter QT interval.

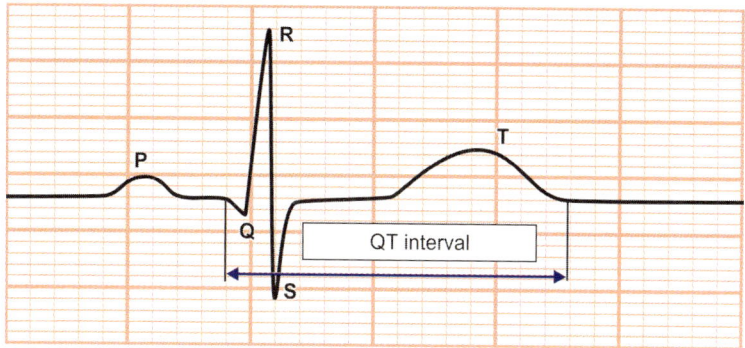

Fig. 5.10: QT interval

- *Bazett's formula* for calculating the heart rate—corrected QT interval (QTc)
- Short QT interval—hypercalcemia
- Increased QT interval—ventricular tachyarrhythmias (torsades de pointes), Jervell syndrome, Lange-Nielsen syndrome, sudden death
- Increased QTc

Hypothyroidism	Older patients	Short stature
Acute hypocalcemia	High systolic blood pressure	Females
During sleep	Acute myocarditis	Acute myocardial infarction
Cerebral injury	Hypothermia	Complete AV block

- Drug-induced increased QT

Haloperidol	Sertindole	High blood alcohol
Vemurafenib	Amiodarone	Thiazide
Ziprasidone	Sotalol	Macrolides
Methadone	Astemizole	Quinidine
Procainamide	Tricyclic antidepressents	

- Short QTc

Digitalis effect	Hypercalcemia	Hyperthermia
Vagal stimulation	Congenital short QT syndrome	

U wave

- Not commonly seen.
- Normal in young children and athletics.
- Follows the T wave.
- Seen in lead V3.
- It is a small wave.
- It represents repolarization of the Purkinje fibers.

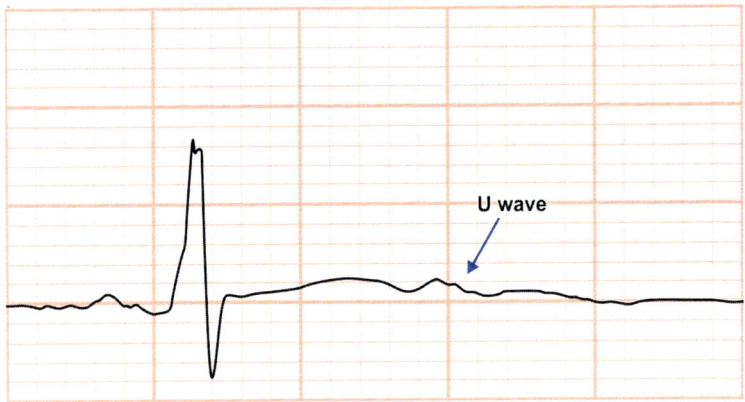

Fig. 5.11: U wave

- Prominent U wave

Hypokalemia	Digitalis	Congenital long QT syndrome
Hypercalcemia	Epinephrine	Intracranial hemorrhage
Thyrotoxicosis	Class 1A and 3 antiarrhythmics	

- Inverted U wave

Myocardial ischemia   Left ventricular volume overload
Left anterior descending coronary artery disease

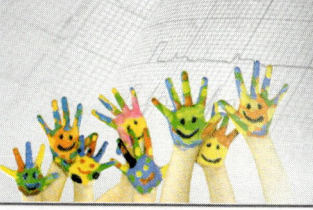

6

Neonatal Electrocardiograph

- Birth → right ventricle → large and thicker than left ventricle
- Right ventricle has a more physiological stress in utero
- P wave
  - Is a vector indicating the direction of activation.
  - P wave with an axis in the quadrant bordered by 0° and +90°.

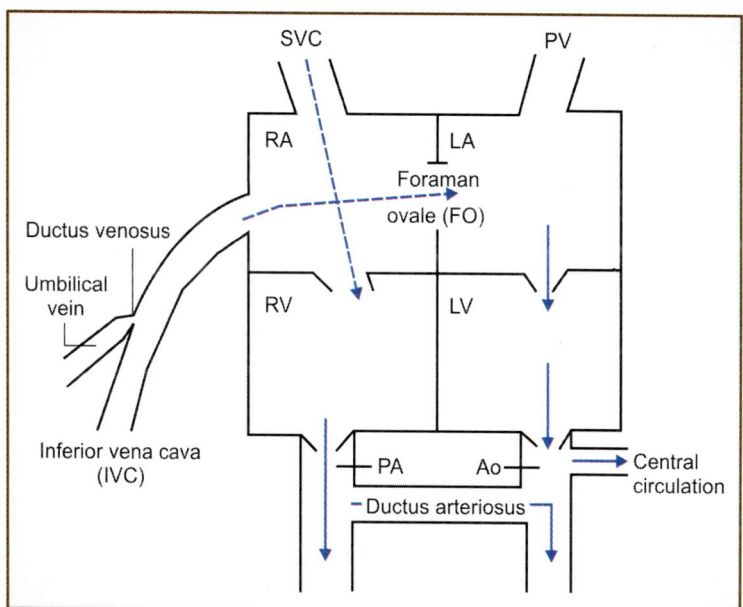

Fig. 6.1: Neonatal cardiac circulation

- Commonly is pointed in lead II and aVF and more rounded in other leads. Lead V1 may be diphasic.
- PR interval
  - PR interval in lead II, increases with age and decreases with heart rate.
  - Normal neonatal PR interval is 70 ms to 140 ms (mean 100 ms.)
- QRS complex
  - Normal full-term neonate has an axis between 55° and 200°.
  - Right axis deviation.
  - In premature newborn it is 65 to 174.
  - QRS duration in the newborn and infant is narrow (<80 ms).
  - Normal QRS duration increases with age.
  - QRS morphology in the newborn may have more notches.
- QT interval
  - Duration changes with rate.
  - Mean QTc on the 4th day of life is 400.
- Others
  - Dominant R wave in V1
  - T-wave inversions in V1–3
  - PR interval, QRS duration—shorter
  - Sinus tachycardia—heart rate goes as high as 180.
  - Right axis deviation +125° +180°.
  - Small voltage—QRS and T waves
  - RV dominance a with tall R waves in V1, V2 and V4R.
  - Benign arrhythmias.
  - Occasional Q waves in V1 (seen in 10% of normal newborns)
  - RV dominance in precordial leads:
    - All R in V1 (>10 mm suggests RVH)
    - Deep S in V6
    - R/S ratio >1 in right chest leads, relatively small in left
  - QRS voltages in limb leads relatively small
  - T waves-low voltage in V1 may be upright for <72 hours (>72 hours suggests RVH).

Preterm Baby

- Shorter QRS duration, shorter PR and QT interval
- Less RV dominance than term infant at birth.

1 Week–1 Month Age

- Right axis retained.
- R waves remain dominant across to V6, although dominant S may be normal
- T wave negative V1
- T wave voltage higher in limb leads.

Normal Values

Age	Ht rate (min)	QRS vector	PR interval sec	QIII mm	QV_6 mm	RV_1 mm
<1 day	93–154	+59 to −163	0.08–0.16	4.5	2	5–26
1–2 days	91–159	+64 to −161	0.08–0.14	6.5	2.5	5–27
3–6 days	91–166	+77 to −163	0.07–0.14	5.5	3	3–24
1–3 weeks	107–182	+65 to −161	0.07–0.14	6	3	3–21

7

Normal Paediatric ECG

- Heart rate >100 beats/min
- Rightward QRS axis
- T wave inversions in V1–3
- Dominant R wave in V1
- RSR′ pattern in V1
- Marked sinus arrhythmia
- Short PR interval (<120 ms)
- Short QRS duration (<80 ms)
- Slightly peaked P waves (<3 mm in height is normal if ≤6 months)
- Slightly long QTc (≤490 ms in infants ≤6 months)
- Q waves in the inferior and left precordial leads.

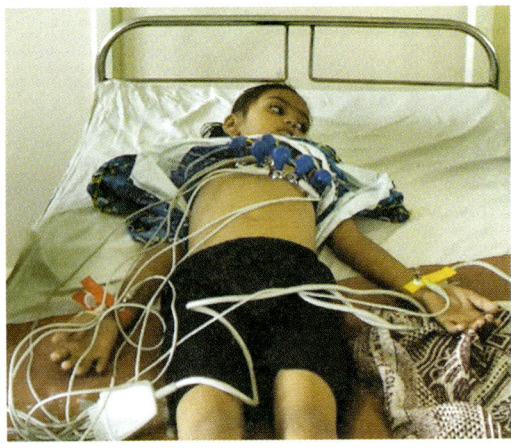

Fig. 7.1: Paediatric ECG

1–6 Months

- QRS axis less than +120°
- R wave dormant in V1
- R/S ratio in V2 close to 1 but may be >1 in V1.
- T waves negative across right chest leads.

6 Months–3 Years

- QRS axis > +90°
- R wave dominant in V6.
- R/S ratio in V1 close to or less than 1.
- Large voltages in precordial leads persist.

3–8 Years

- Adult QRS progression in precordial leads: Dominant S in V1, dominant R in V6.
- Large precordial voltages persist.
- Q waves in left chest leads may be large (<5 mm).
- T waves remain negative in right precordial leads.

8–16 Years

- QRS axis 0° to +90°.
- Adult QRS progression.
- Large precordial lead voltages, R in left lead larger than adult.
- T waves variable. Maybe upright in V1 but negative V1–V4 not abnormal.

Adult

- QRS axis range 0° to +100°
- Dominant LV
- T waves upright across precordial leads.

Indications for Paediatrics Electrocardiography

- Diagnosis and management of congenital heart disease
- Diagnosis and management of arrhythmia
- Diagnosis and management of rheumatic fever, Kawasaki's disease, pericarditis, myocarditis
- Syncope and seizures

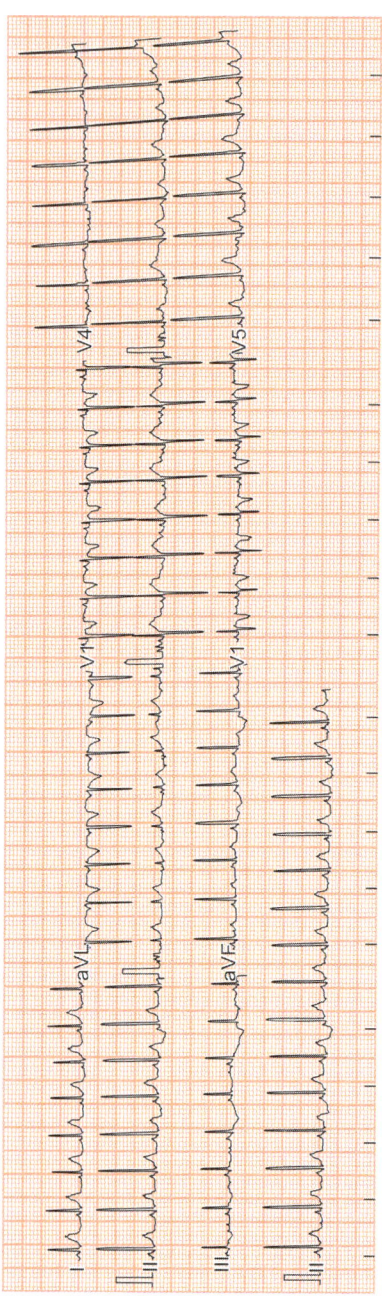

Fig. 7.2: Paediatric ECG

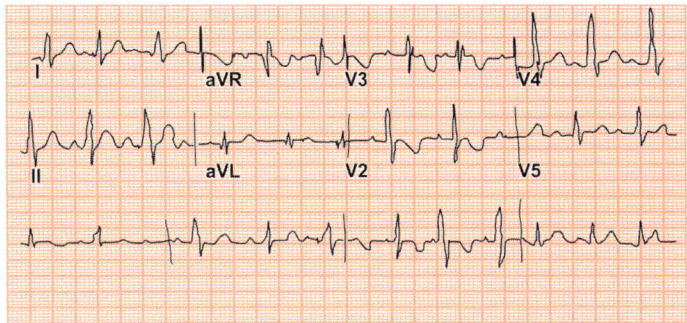

Fig. 7.3: Normal paediatric ECG

- Cyanotic episodes
- Chest pain or exertion-related symptoms
- Family history of sudden death or life-threatening event
- Electrolyte abnormalities
- Drug ingestion.

Evans Rules

- Small chest walls exaggerate precordial voltages.
- Evans, et al. proposed a practical approach to evaluation.
- Abnormal left ventricular large voltage
    - Use only V6 (left most precordial lead).
    - If R wave of V6 intersects with baseline of V5—abnormal
- Abnormal right ventricular large voltage
- Use only V1 (rightmost precordial lead)
    - Upright T wave in V1: In first week of life is normal. Between week 1 and adolescence—abnormal
    - RSR′ in V1: If R′ is taller than R—abnormal.
    - Pure R wave in V1: If child > 6 months old—abnormal.

Normal ECG Findings in Athletic Children

1. Sinus bradycardia
2. Sinus arrhythmia
3. Ectopic atrial rhythm
4. Junctional escape rhythm
5. First degree AV block (PR interval > 200 msec)
6. Mobitz type I (Wenckebach) 2° AV block
7. Incomplete RBBB.

8

Cardiac Chamber Enlargement

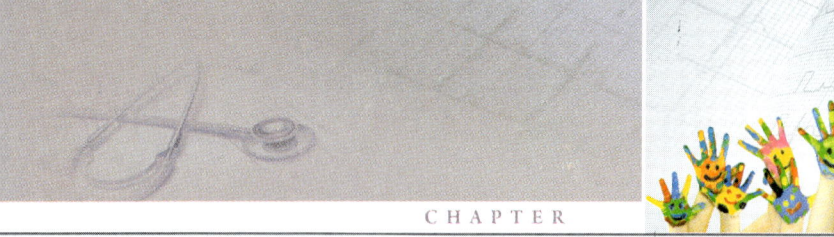

Left Atrial Enlargement

- Prolongation of terminal component of atrial activation
- Posterior deviation of left atrial vector
- Lead V1—broad P wave (>0.04 sec or 1 small square)
- Deeply negative P wave (>1 mm) terminal
- Leads I and II—P wave duration >0.12 sec
- Left atrial enlargement—mitral valve insufficiency.

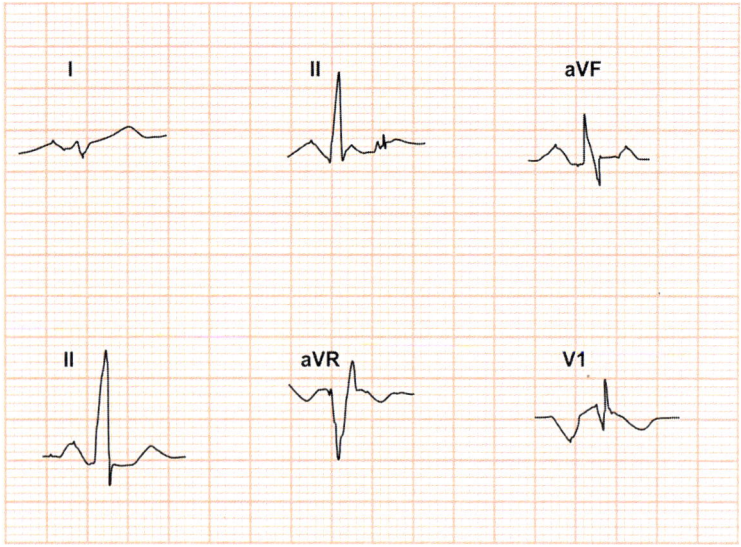

Fig. 8.1: Left atrial enlargement

Right Atrial Enlargement

- Lead II, III, aVF—P wave: >2.5 mm
- Lead V1—P wave: >1.5 mm
- P wave: Positive part of biphasic wave is larger than negative part.
- P congenital may be present.
- Right atrial enlargement-after pulmonary embolization.

Biatrial Enlargement

Biphasic P Wave

- More than 0.04 sec duration in lead V1
- Positive initial part is >1.5 mm.
- Negative terminal part >1 mm.
- Wide and notched P wave in frontal plane leads.

Causes

- Mitral stenosis associated marked pulmonary hypertension
- Mitral stenosis associated with tricuspid regurgitation
- Mitral stenosis associated with tricuspid stenosis
- Atrial septal defect
- Lutembacher's syndrome.

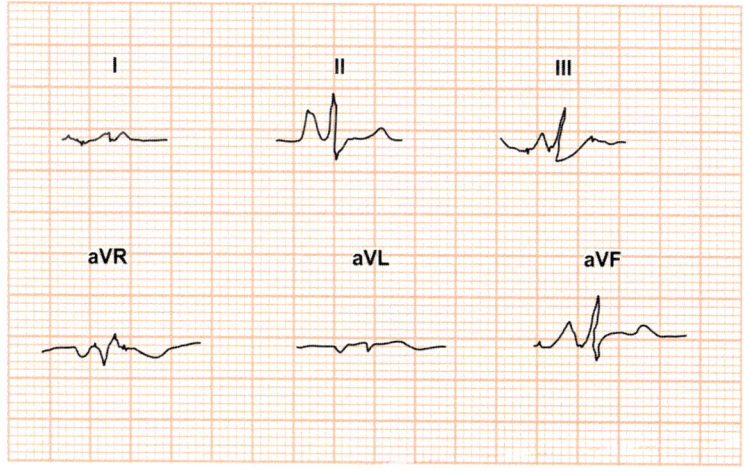

Fig. 8.2: Right atrial enlargement

LVH

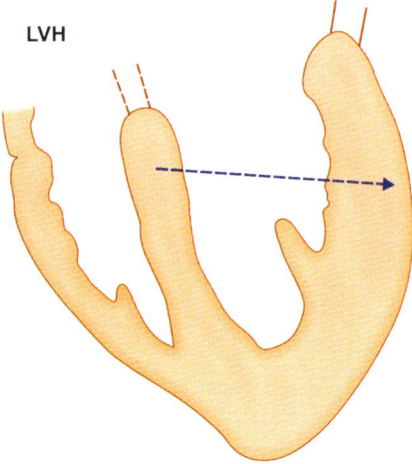

Fig. 8.3: Left ventricular hypertrophy

Left Ventricular Hypertrophy

- Results from an increase in left ventricular workload—systolic and diastolic overload.
- Systolic overload is due to aortic stenosis, systemic hypertension, hypertrophic cardiomyopathy, coartaction of aorta.
- Diastolic overload is due to patent ductus arteriosus, ventricular septal defect.
- ECG changes in systolic overload
    - Increased magnitude of QRS deflections
    - Increased QRS systolic overload duration
    - Counter clockwise electrical rotation
    - Increase in left ventricular activation time
    - Attenuation of small Q wave
    - Abnormalities of the ST segment and T wave
    - Inversion of U wave in left precordial leads.
- ECG changes in diastolic overload
    - Tall R wave in left leads
    - Deep narrow Q wave left leads
    - Tall symmetrical T wave
    - Minimally elevated ST segment in left leads
    - Inverted U waves in left leads.

- Causes
  - Hypertension
  - Aortic valve stenosis

ECG Changes

- Leads V1–V6: Large QRS complex.
- Lead V1—deep S wave
- Lead V4–lead V1
- Leads V5–V6: ST depression
- Sokolow-Lyon criteria
  - For diagnosis of LVH, above the age of 40 years
  - R in V5 or V6 in mm + S in V1 in mm—>35 mm
  - 10–29 year—99th percentile for SV1+RV5 is 53 mm
- Cornell criterion
  - Male—R in aVL and S in V3 >28 mm
  - Female—R in aVL and S in V3 >20 mm

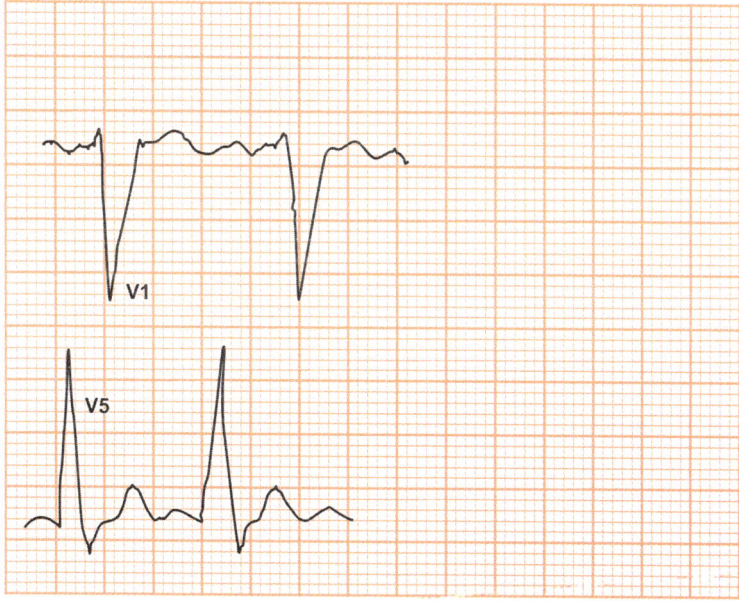

Fig. 8.4: Left ventricular hypertrophy

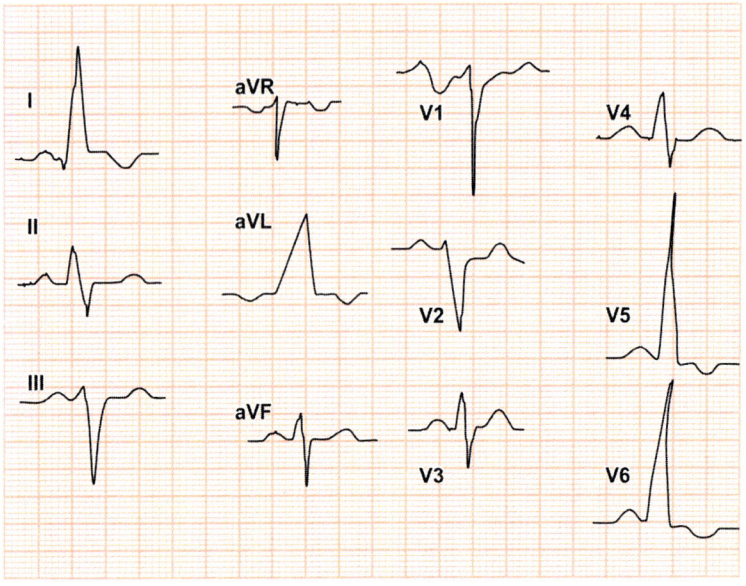

Fig. 8.5: Left ventricular hypertrophy

Right Ventricular Hypertrophy

- Results from an increase in right ventricular workload.
- Causes
  - Emphysema
  - Pulmonary embolization
  - Congenital heart disease

ECG Changes

- Lead I—negative QRS complex
- Right axis deviation
- Dominance of R wave in right leads
- Lead V1—positive QRS complex in V1
- QRS duration <120 ms
- Lead V1—intrinsicoid deflections
- Right bundle branch block
- Dominant R wave:
  - R/S ratio in V1 or V3R >1
  - R/S ratio in V5 or V6 ≤1

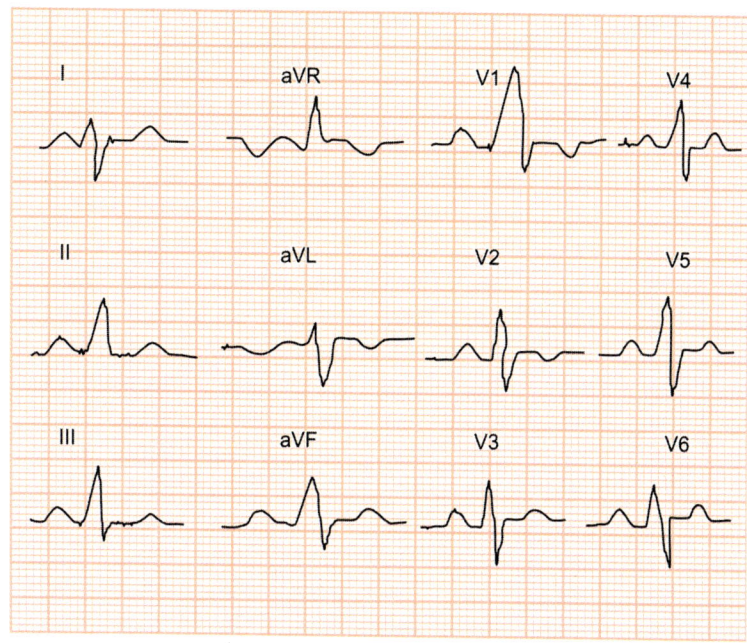

Fig. 8.6: Right ventricular hypertrophy

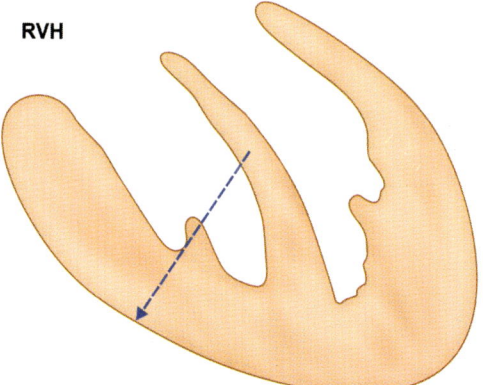

Fig. 8.7: Right ventricular hypertrophy

– R wave in V1 ≥7 mm
– R wave in V1 + S wave in V5 or V6 >10.5 mm

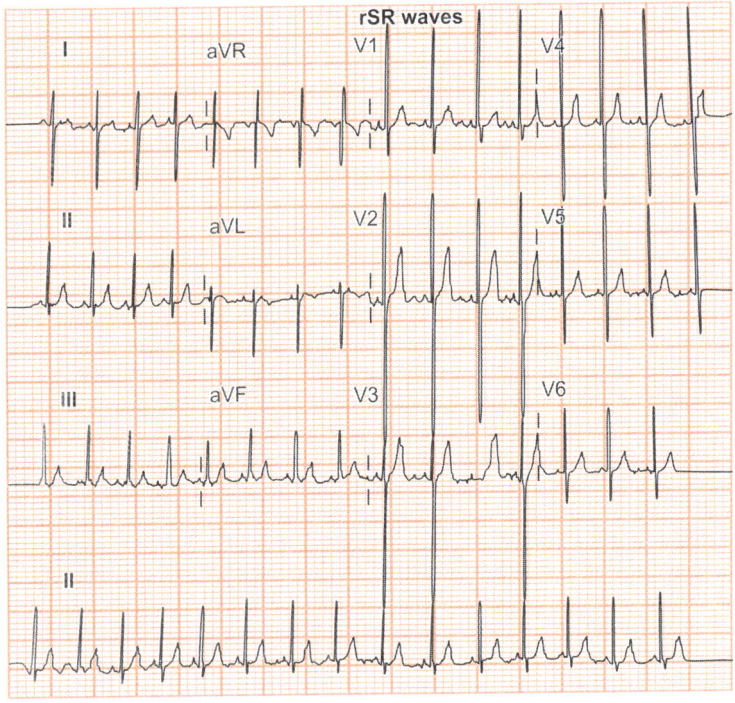

Fig. 8.8: rSR ECG

– rSR—in V1 with R′—>10 mm
– qR complex in V1

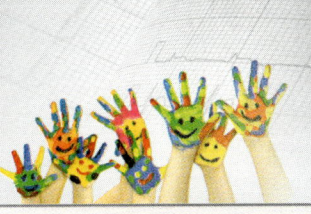

9

Bundle Branch Block

Right Bundle Branch Block

A delay or block of conduction within the right bundle branch.

- Complete RBBB
  - Duration of QRS >120
  - V1—rSR pattern.
  - Lead 1 and V6—slurred S wave.
  - Lead V1—tall, wide and frequently notched R wave.
  - Lead V5 and V6—prominent, delayed and widened S wave in
  - Small r wave
- Incomplete RBBB
  - Duration of QRS—100 to 120
  - Diminuation of S wave in lead V2
  - Small r deflection in lead V2
  - rsr' configuration

Left Bundle Branch Block

- Due to delay or interruption of conduction within the left bundle branch.
- LBBB indicates underlying heart disease, acute myocardial infarction, left ventricular dysfunction
- Complete LBBB
  - Duration of QRS is >120 ms
  - Delay and anomalous activation of left septal mass
  - Tall and notched R wave

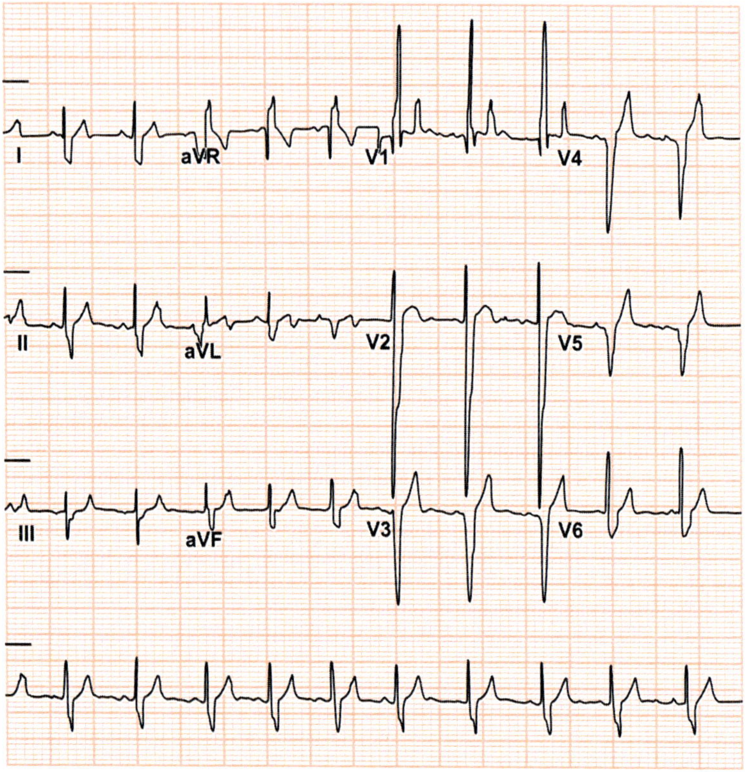

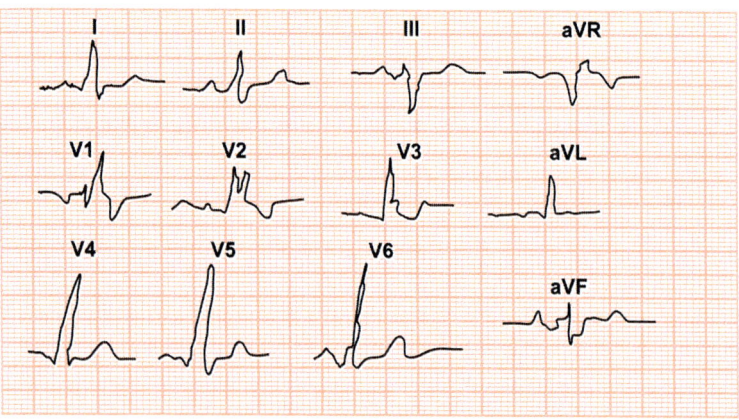

Fig. 9.1: Right bundle branch block

Fig. 9.2: Right bundle branch block

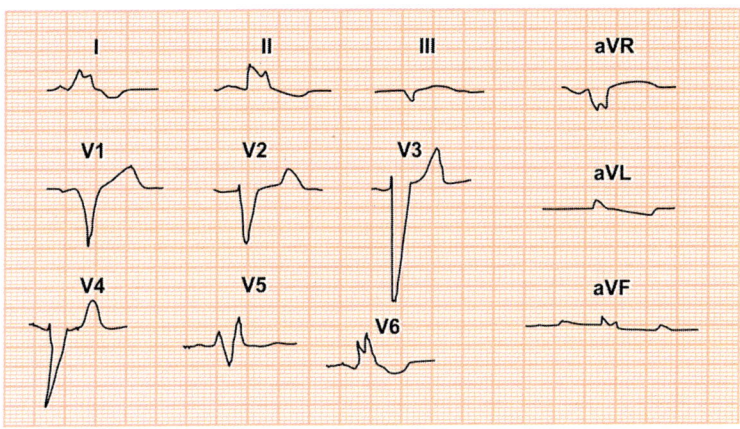

Fig. 9.3: Left bundle branch block

- Lead V1, V2: Widened and notched QS
- Lead V2: Small initial r wave
- ST segment and T wave are opposite in direction in QRS deflection
- Lead V6: Wide RR' deflection.
- rS complexes-small initial r wave with deep and wide S wave.
- Lead V5 and V6: Depressed ST segment.
- Lead V1, V2: Asymmetrical T wave.
- Incomplete LBBB
  - Duration of QRS is 100–120 ms
  - Single, tall R wave
  - Small initial Q wave in lead V5, V6
  - Small initial r wave in lead V1.

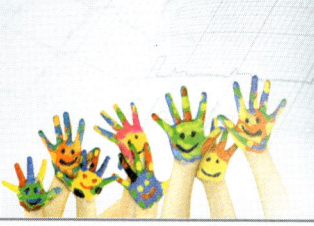

10

Congenital Acyanotic Heart Diseases

Atrial Septal Defect

- Congenital acyanotic heart defect.
- 1 child per 1500 live births.
- Left to right shunt.
- Communication through interatrial septum.
- Oxygenrich blood flows directly from left atrium to right atrium of heart.

Causes

Down syndrome	Ebstein's anomaly	Fetal alcohol syndrome
Holt-Oram syndrome	Lutembacher's syndrome	

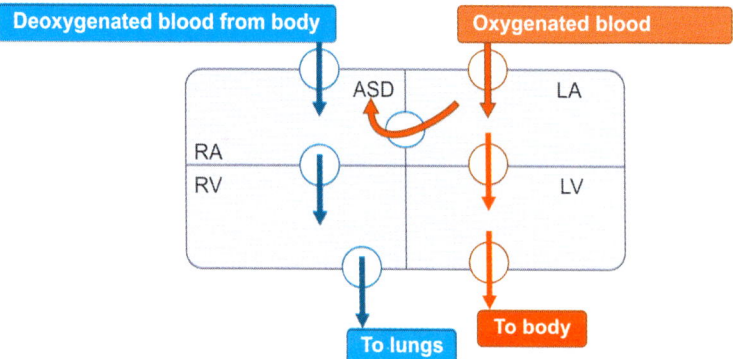

Fig. 10.1: Atrial septal defect

Clinical Features

- Pulmonary systolic ejection murmur
- Second heart sound—fixed splitting.

Ostium Secundum ASD

- Most common
- 6–10% of all congenital heart diseases
- Arises from an enlarged foramen ovale
- Asso with mitral valve prolapse
- Lutembacher's syndrome—ostium secundum ASD + acquired mitral valve stenosis.
- Do not have significant symptoms through early adulthood.

Clinical Features

Exercise intolerance tolerance	Easy fatigability
Palpitations	Syncope

Complications

Pulmonary hypertension	Right-sided heart failure	Atrial fibrillation
Atrial flutter	Stroke	Eisenmenger's syndrome (5 to 10%)

Patent Foramen Ovale

- A remnant of the fetal foramen ovale
- Normally closes at birth
- 25%
- Common in patients with atrial septal
- Surgical closure
- Percutaneous device closure
- Anticoagulant and antiplatelet treatment

Ostium Primum ASD (Atrioventricular Septal Defect)

- Less common
- Usually associated with down syndrome.

Electrocardiogram

- Prolonged PR interval

- Primum ASD—left axis deviation of the QRS complex
- Secundum ASD—right axis deviation of the QRS complex.

Secundum Atrial Septal Defect

- Normal sinus rhythm

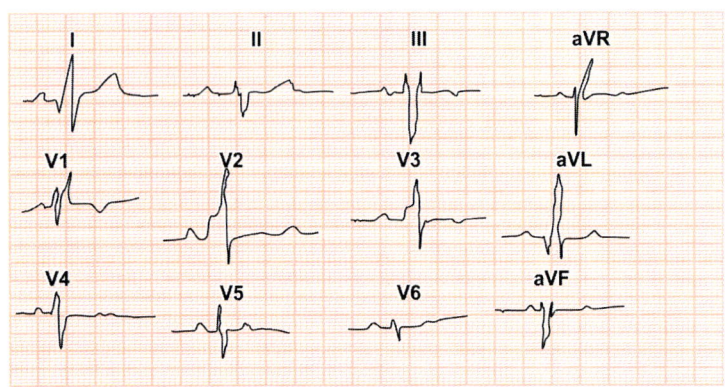

Fig. 10.2: Ostium primum ASD

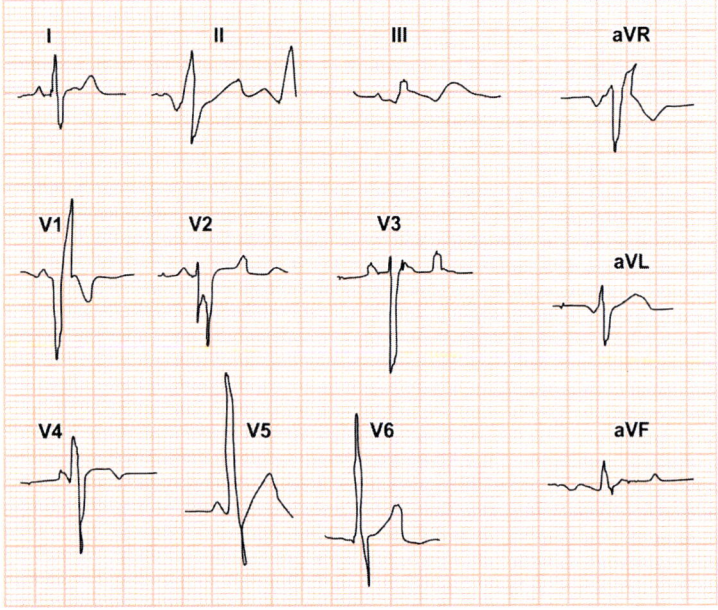

Fig. 10.3: Ostium secundum ASD

- PR interval—first degree AV block
- QRS axis—right axis deviation (0° to 180°)
- QRS configuration: rSr′ or rsR′
- Right atrial enlargement
- 'Crochetage' pattern

Large Ostium Primum Defect with Dilated Right Heart

Ventricular Septal Defect

- Most common congenital cardiac abnormalities
- 2–6 per 1000 births
- Acyanotic congenital heart defect
- Left-to-right shunt
- Defect in the ventricular septum, between left and right ventricles of the heart.

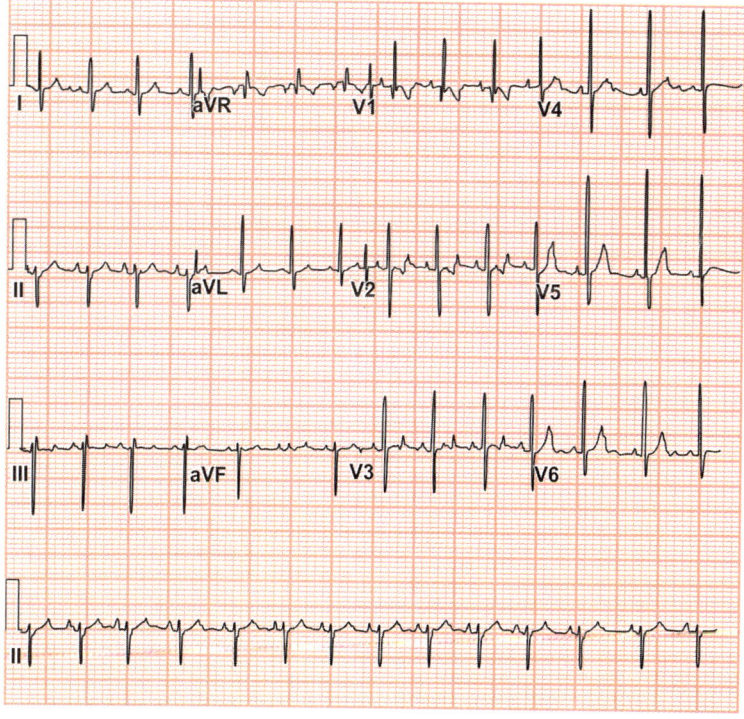

Fig. 10.4: Ventricular septal defect

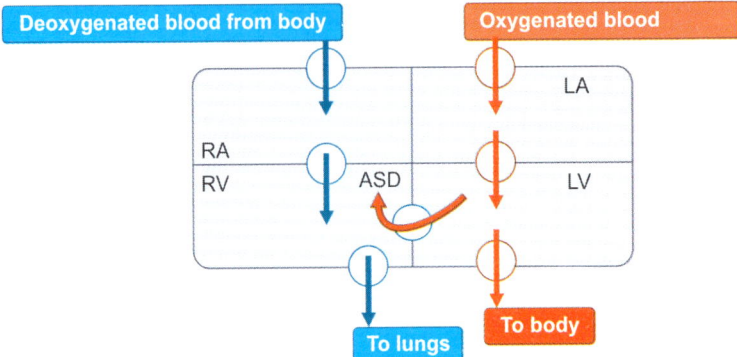

Fig. 10.5: Ventricular septal defect

- Ventricular contraction (systole) → blood → left ventricle → leaks → right ventricle → lungs → pulmonary veins → left atrium → left ventricle
- Left ventricle volume overload → increased right ventricular pressure → pulmonary hypertension
- Congenital VSD—Down syndrome
- Types of VSD

Perimembranous (common)	Outlet
Atrioventricular	Muscular (rare)

- Usually symptomless at birth
- Manifests a few weeks after birth
- Pansystolic (holosystolic) murmur along lower left sternal border
- Normal heart sounds
- Displaced apex beat
- Small VSD-louder murmur and palpable thrill
- Larger VSD
  - Fail to thrive
  - Sweaty
  - Tachypnea during feeds
  - Parasternal heave
  - Associated with pulmonary hypertension

- Eisenmenger's syndrome
  - Large VSD
  - VSD becomes a right-to-left shunt
  - Increased pressures in the pulmonary vascular bed.
- ECG
  - Small VSD—normal
  - Moderately restrictive VSD—left atrial enlargement
  - Swiss cheese ventricular septum, ventricular septal aneurysms, moderately restrictive VSD, inlet VSDs and AV septal defects: Left axis deviation.
  - Large VSD—biventricular enlargement-Katz-Wachtel phenomenon—tall diphasic RS complexes at least 50 mm in height in lead V2, V3 or V4—mid-precordial leads.

Patent Ductus Arteriosus

- 1:2000 births at term
- Common in females
- More in premature babies
- Association with congenital rubella, maternal warfarin treatment.
- Ductus arteriosus connects aorta to the pulmonary artery.
- Aortic pressure > pulmonary artery.
- Shunt flow is from aorta → pulmonary artery.
- Increased blood flow → left atrium → left ventricle.
- Blood flows into pulmonary artery in both systole and diastole causing continuous murmur.
- Increased pulmonary flow → decreases lung compliance.

Clinical Features

Asymptomatic	Premature babies with respiratory disease
Failure to thrive	Cyanosis ? Eisenmenger syndrome
Cardiorespiratory failure	Machinery continuous flow murmur below left clavicle
Right ventricular heave	Loud P2
Increased pulse volume	Mid diastolic flow murmur at apex

- ECG
  - Small PDA—normal

- Moderate PDA—left atrial abnormality, left ventricular hypertrophy.
- Large PDA—biventricular hypertrophy pattern, prolongation of PR interval, deep S wave in V1
- Tall R waves in V5 and V6.
- Normal sinus rhythm
- Normal QRS axis
- Left atrial enlargement

Coarctation of Aorta

- 'Coarctation' means narrowing.
- Congenital condition
- Aorta is narrow at the ductus arteriosus (ligamentum arteriosum after regression).
- Common in the aortic arch
- Types of aortic coarctations

1. Preductal coarctation:
   - Proximal to the ductus arteriosus
   - Seen in 5% of infants with Turner syndrome
2. Ductal coarctation: At the insertion of the ductus arteriosus.
3. Postductal coarctation:
   - Most common
   - Seen at distal to the insertion of the ductus arteriosus
   - Associated with notching of the ribs
   - Hypertension in the upper extremities

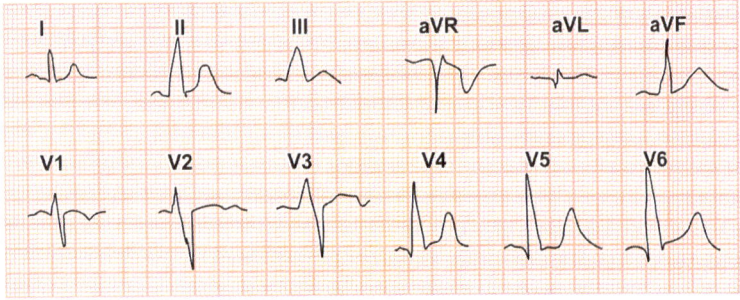

Fig. 10.6: Patent ductus arteriosus

- Weak pulses in the lower extremities
- Arterial hypertension in the arms
- Low blood pressure in the lower extremities.

Clinical Features

Mild—no signs or symptoms	Twice common in boys	Girls—Turner syndrome
Difficulty breathing	Poor appetite	Failure to thrive
Dizziness	Shortness of breath	Fainting episodes
Chest pain	Fatigue	Headaches
Nose bleeds	Cold legs and feet	Pain in legs with exercise (intermittent claudication)

- X-ray—poststenotic dilatation of the aorta results in a classic 'figure 3 sign' on
- ECG
  - Normal sinus rhythm
  - Normal PR interval

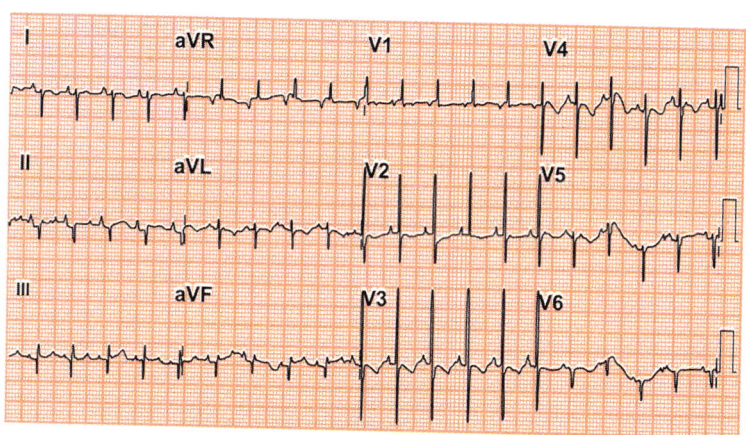

Fig. 10.7: Coarctation of aorta

- Normal or left axis deviation
- Normal QRS configuration
- Left atrial enlargement
- Left ventricular hypertrophy.

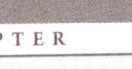

11

Congenital Cyanotic Heart Diseases

Pulmonic Stenosis

- Congenital malformation of the pulmonary valve.
- Valve orifice fails to develop.
- Obstructing the outflow of blood from the heart to the lungs.
- Types
    1. Pulmonary atresia with intact ventricular septum—rare, complete blockage of the pulmonary valve.
    2. Pulmonary atresia with ventricular septal defect—under development of the right ventricle.
- Features—cyanosis, fatigue, shortness of breath
- Associated defects—tricuspid atresia, tetralogy of Fallot, RVw/double outlet.

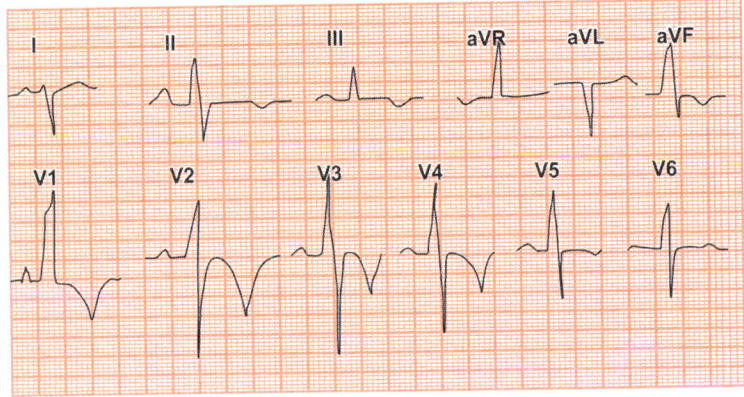

Fig. 11.1: Pulmonic stenosis

- ECG changes
  - Normal sinus rhythm
  - Normal PR interval
  - QRS axis: Normal if mild; RAD with moderate/severe
  - rSr' pattern
  - Right atrial enlargement
  - Right ventricular hypertrophy.

Ebstein's Anomaly

- Huge P waves
- Low amplitude QRS wave
- T wave inversion
- Normal sinus rhythm
- QRS axis: Normal or LAD
- Right atrial enlargement

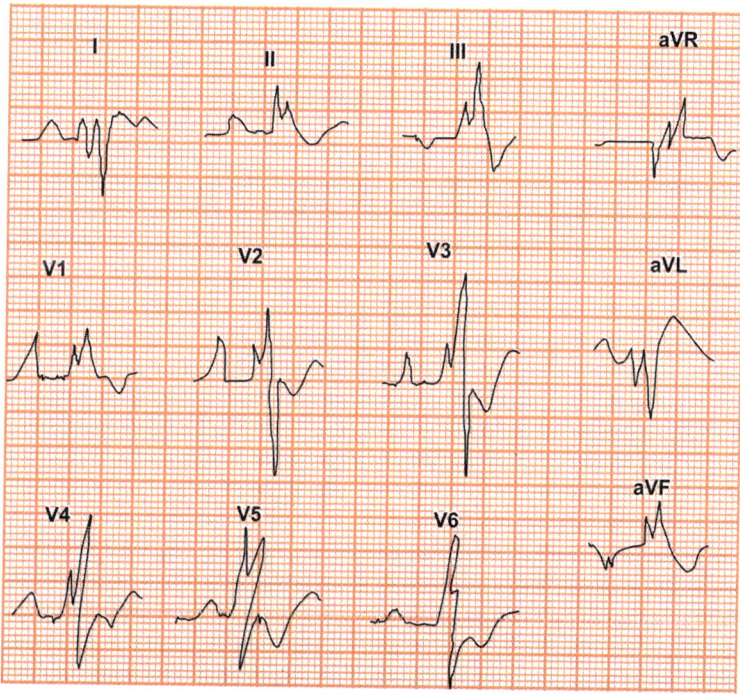

Fig. 11.2: Ebstein's anomaly

Tetralogy of Fallot

- 7 to 10% of all congenital heart abnormalities
- 1 in 2,000 newborns
- Most common complex congenital heart defect
- Right-to-left shunt
- Described in 1671 by Niels Stensen
- 1888: Detailed description by French physician Étienne-Louis Arthur Fallot.
- Maternal risk factors

Use of alcohol	Rubella during pregnancy
Maternal diabetes	Associated with Down syndrome
Age over 40	

- Four defects:
  - Ventricular septal defect
  - Pulmonary stenosis
  - Right ventricular hypertrophy
  - Overriding of aorta
- Clinical features

Cyanotic nail beds	Heart murmur
Difficulty in feeding	Failure to gain weight
Retarded growth and development	Dyspnea on exertion
Clubbing of the fingers and toes	Polycythemia

- Tet spells/cyanotic spells—sudden, marked increase in cyanosis → syncope → hypoxic brain injury → death.

Acute hypoxia spells	Shortness of breath
Cyanosis	Agitation
Loss of consciousness	Squat

- Chest X-ray
  - Coeur-en-sabot
  - Boot-like heart
  - Absence of interstitial lung markings
  - Pulmonary oligaemia
- ECG
  - Tall R waves in V1
  - Prominent P waves in V1

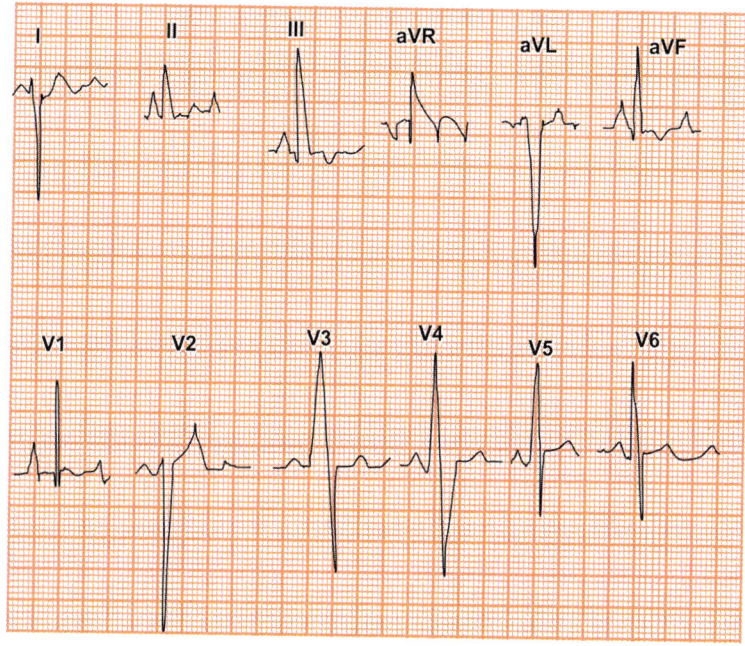

Fig. 11.3: Tetralogy of Fallot

- Rightward deviated axis
- Abnormal R/S ratio in V1
- Abnormally low R/S ratio in V6
- Abnormally deep S waves in V6
- Abnormal R wave in V1
- Abnormal T wave in the right precordium and Q waves in V1.

Surgically Repaired TOF

- Normal sinus rhythm
- PR interval: Normal or mild ↑
- Peaked P waves
- QRS axis: Normal or RAD; LAD (5–10%)
- RBBB
- Right atrial enlargement
- Right ventricular hypertrophy

Total Anomalous Pulmonary Venous Connection

- Rare cyanotic congenital heart defect
- All four pulmonary veins are malpositioned
- Anomalous connections to the systemic venous circulation
- Fatal condition
- Lack of systemic blood flow
- Types—supracardiac, cardiac and infra-diaphragmatic
- Clinical features

Right ventricular heave	Systolic ejection murmur at left upper sternal border
Loud S1	Cardiomegaly
Fixed split S2	Right axis deviation
S3 gallop	Right ventricular hypertrophy
Tachypnea, dyspnea, cyanosis	Cottage-loaf sign-chest X-ray 'snow man' sign or 'figure of 8' sign

- ECG changes
  - Sinus bradycardia
  - Normal PR interval
  - Right axis deviation
  - Absence of q, small r, deep S in left precordium
  - Right atrial enlargement
  - Right ventricular hypertrophy

Congenitally Corrected TGA

- Also known as levo-transposition of the great arteries.
- Acynotic congenital heart defect.
- Aorta and pulmonary artery are transposed.
- Aortais anterior and to the left of the pulmonary artery.
- Corresponding atrioventricular valves are also transposed.
- Ventricular inversion.
- Deoxygenated blood → right atrium → left ventricle (lies on right side of heart) → pulmonary artery → lungs → oxygenated blood → pulmonary veins → left atrium → morphological right ventricle → aorta.
- ECG
  - Normal sinus rhythm
  - PR interval

- Left axis deviation
- Absence Q in III, aVF, and right precordium.

Aortic Stenosis

- Common valvular heart disease.
- 1663—first described by French physician Lazare Rivière.
- Narrowing of the exit of the left ventricle of the heart where the aorta begins.
- It may be at, above or below aortic valve.
- Causes

Acute rheumatic fever	Fabry disease
Systemic lupus erythematosus	Paget disease
High blood uric acid levels	Infection

- Clinical features

Heart failure	Loss of consciousness
Chest pain	Shortness of breath
Swelling of the legs	Pallor with a light flush
Angina	Syncope

- Complications—endocarditis and syncope
- Cardiac findings
    - Low volume pulse
    - *Pulsus parvus et tardus*
    - Apical-carotid delay
    - Ejection click at lower left sternal border and apex
    - Systolic, crescendo-decrescendo murmur (upper right sternal border)
    - Decreased and softer second heart sound
    - Audible fourth heart sound
- Electrocardiogram
    - Left ventricular hypertrophy
    - Left bundle branch block

Hypoplastic Left Heart Syndrome

- Rare congenital heart defect.
- Left side of heart is severely underdeveloped.

- Aorta and left ventricle are also underdeveloped.
- Aortic and mitral valves are either too small to allow sufficient blood flow or are atretic.
- Blood returns from the lungs to the left atrium and passes through atrial septal defect to the right side of the heart.
- Dangerously low circulation → shock
- Cyanotic at birth.
- Associated syndromes

Trisomy 13 (Patau syndrome)	Jacobsen syndrome
Trisomy 18 (Edwards syndrome)	Holt-Oram syndrome
Partial Trisomy 9	Smith-Lemli-Opitz syndrome
Turner's syndrome	

- ECG changes
  - Right ventricular hypertrophy
  - Diminished left ventricular forces
  - Absent Q waves in the lateral precordial leads
  - Longer PR interval
  - A wider QRS complex.

Transposition of the Great Vessels

- 1797—first described by Matthew Baillie.
- Dextro-transposition of the great arteries—deoxygenated blood → right heart → aorta → body (bypassing the lungs) is cyanotic.
- Levo-transposition of the great arteries—acyanotic, systemic and the pulmonary circulation are connected.
- chest X-ray—egg on a string
- ECG changes
  - Tall and peaked P waves
  - Right ventricular hypertrophy
  - Rightward shift of frontal plane of QRS axis.

Tricuspid Atresia

- Congenital heart disease
- Complete absence of the tricuspid valve
- Absence of right atrioventricular connection

- Hypoplastic or absent right ventricle
- Clinical manifestations
  - Progressive cyanosis
  - Poor feeding
  - Tachypnea
  - Holosystolic murmur due to the VSD
- ECG
  - Left axis deviation
  - Left ventricular hypertrophy

Eissenmenger's Syndrome

- Tardive cyanosis
- 1897—Dr Victor Eisenmenger, who first described.
- Long-standing left-to-right cardiac shunt.
- Ventricular septal defect, atrial septal defect, or patent ductus arteriosus → pulmonary hypertension.
- Reversal of the shunt into a cyanotic right-to-left shunt
- Features

Cyanosis	Clubbing
Syncope	Heart failure
Endocarditis	Pneumonia
Stroke	Gout
Gallstones	

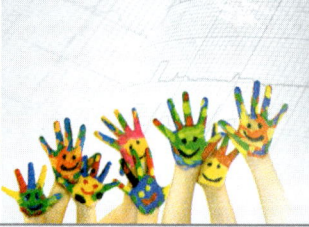

12

Dextrocardia/Situs Inversus

Dextrocardia

- Apex of the heart is directed towards the right side of the chest.
- ECG findings
  - Predominantly negative P wave, QRS complex, and T wave in lead I.
  - Low voltage in leads V3–V6
  - Inversion of P waves in leads I and Avl
  - Dominant S waves in leads I and V1 to V6
  - Reversed R wave progression in chest leads
  - Low voltage QRS axis in V4 to V6
  - Extreme QRS axis
  - Flattened T waves in V4 to V6 and aVR
  - Inverted T waves in lead I and aVL.

Dextrocardia with Situs Inversus

Abnormal positioning of the heart and other internal organs.

Situs Inversus

- Mirror image reversal of the organs in the chest and abdominal cavity.
- ECG changes
  - Normal sinus rhythm
  - P-wave axis—105° to 165°
  - Normal PR interval

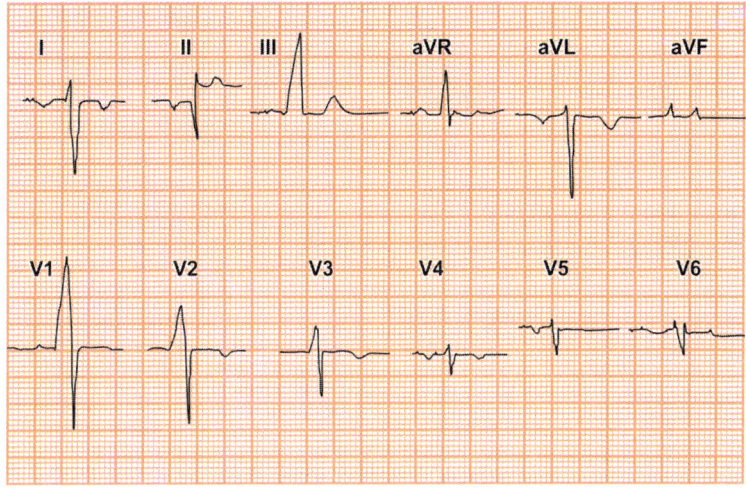

Fig. 12.1: Dextrocardia

- Right axis deviation
- QRS configuration: Inverse depolarization and repolarization
- Left ventricular hypertrophy—tall R in V1–V2
- Right ventricular hypertrophy—deep Q, small R in V1 and tall R in right lateral leads.

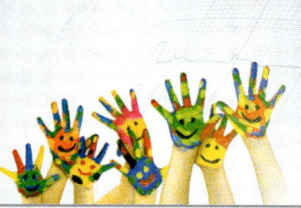

13

Carditis in Children

Pericarditis

- Inflammation of the pericardium
- QRS voltages less than 5 mm in all limb leads.
- Acute pericarditis
  - Infective, autoimmune, neoplastic, radiation injury or metabolic causes.
  - Elevated concave—upwards ST segments or saddle shaped appearance of ST segment
  - ST segment axis +30° to +60°
  - J point elevation
  - Early: T wave slightly taller, peaked
  - Later on T wave inversion
  - Early PTa wavein opposite direction of P wave
  - PR segment depression with upright P wave
  - In lead aVR and V1 PR segment elevation with inverted P wave
  - No changes in QRS complex
  - Sinus tachycardia

Myocarditis

- PR prolongation to complete AV dissociation
- Low QRS voltages
- Increased QRS duration
- QRS complex lose their smooth outline
- Pathological Q waves

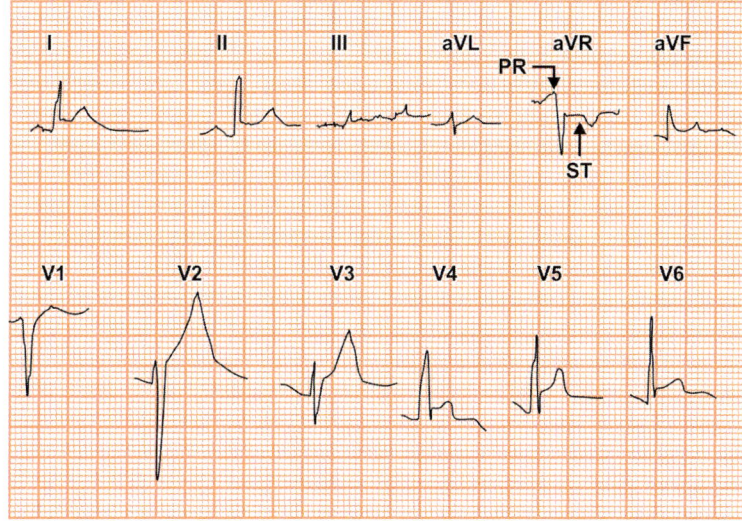

Fig. 13.1: Acute pericarditis

- Loss of r wave amplitude
- ST segment may be elevated or depressed
- Decreased T wave amplitude
- Low to inverted T wave in left oriented leads
- QT prolongation
- Tachyarrhythmias including SVT and VT
- First degree AV block
- 'Pseudoinfarction' pattern with deep Q waves and poor R wave progression in precordial leads.
- Sinus tachycardia

Myocardial Infarction

- Rare in children
- Cellular damage due to prolonged ischaemia
- Infarction: ST elevation in contiguous leads with reciprocal ST depression elsewhere
- Ischaemia: Horizontal ST depression
- Development of new pathological Q waves
- Presence of ST segment elevation or depresentation
- Development of new LBBB

- Tall, symmetrical, peaked and widened T waves
- Slope elevation of ST segment
- Increased amplitude of R wave
- Increased ventricular activation time
- Appearance of new Q wave in the form of QS, Qr, Qr
- Decrease in R wave height
- J point and ST elevation in acute phase
- Tall peaked T wave in acute phase
- Prolongation of QT interval
- Sclarovsky-Birnbaum score
- Grade 1: Tall, symmetrical, peaked and widened T waves
- Grade 2: Slope elevation of ST segment
- Grade 3: Distortion of terminal QRS complex

14

Electrolyte Imbalance

Hypocalcemia

- Prolongation of ST segment
- prolongation of QTc
- P wave, QRS complex and U wave are unaffected.
- Prolongation of QT interval is inversely proportional to the serum calcium level.

Hypercalcemia

- Marked shortening of QT interval
- Shortens the ST segment
- T wave is relatively unaffected.

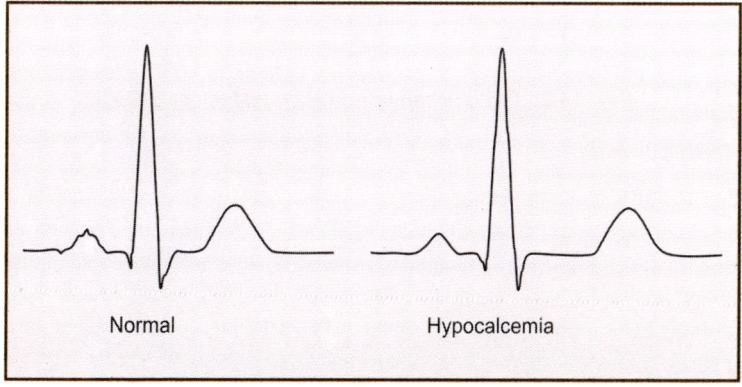

Fig. 14.1: Hypocalcemia

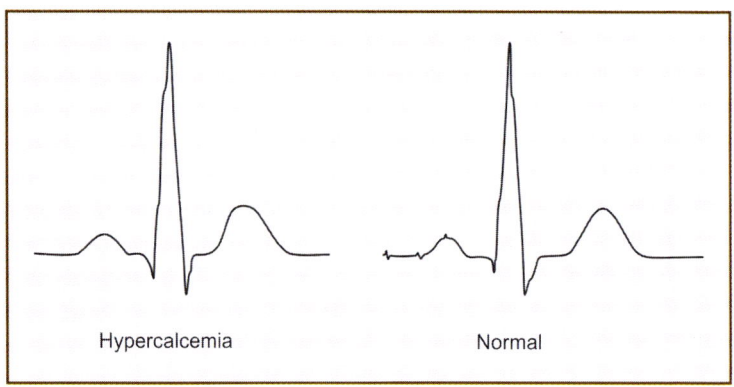

Fig. 14.2: Hypercalcemia

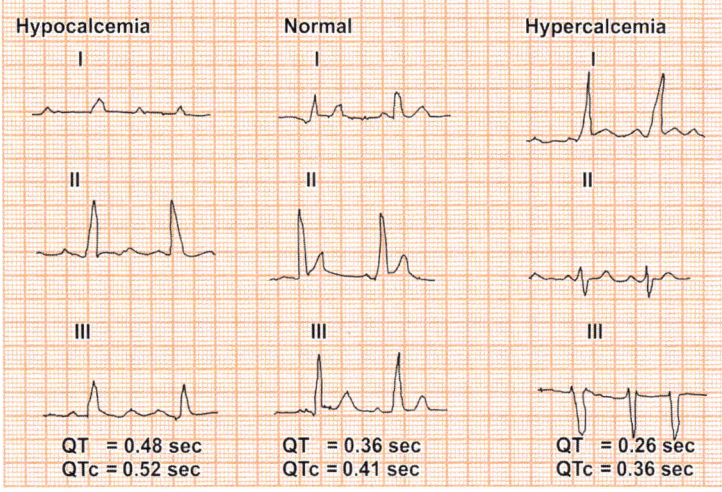

Fig. 14.3: Hypocalcemia and hypercalcemia ECG

Hypokalemia

- Prominent U waves
- Prolongation of the QTc
- Flat or biphasic T waves
- ST segment depression
- Prolonged PR interval
- Sinoatrial block
- Progressive diminuation of T wave

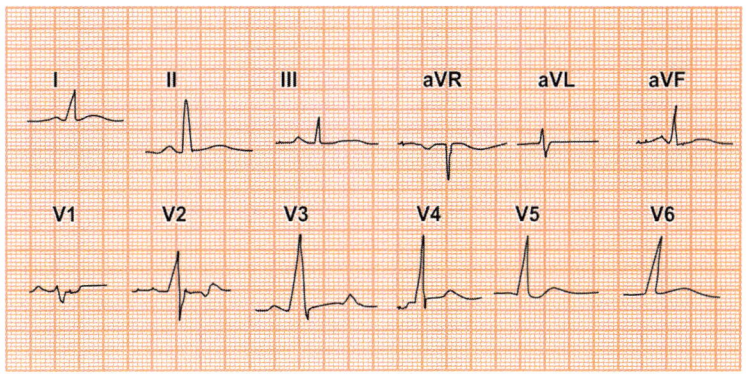

Fig. 14.4: Hypokalemia ECG

- Progressive increase of ampltitude of U wave
- First and second degree AV block

Hyperkalemia

- Tall peaked T waves, best seen in precordial leads
- Prolongation of QRS duration
- Prolongation of PR interval
- Disappearance of P waves
- Wide bizarre biphasic QRS complexes (sine waves)
- Eventual asystole

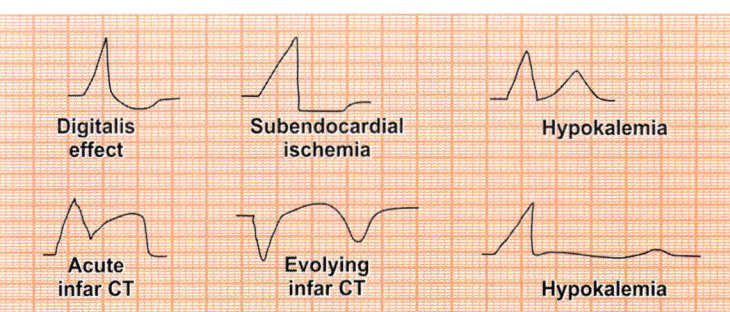

Fig. 14.5: ECG in various conditions

- Virtual disappearance of ST segment
- QT interval normal/decreased
- Any degree of AV block.

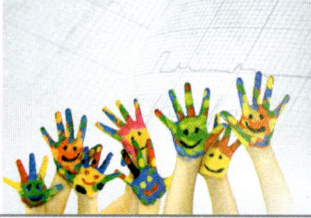

15

Cardiac Arrhythmias

Atrial Fibrillation

- Most common sustained cardiac arrhythmia
- Occurs in mitral and tricuspid valvular disease, coronary artery disease, hypertension, hyperthyroidism.
- Excitation and recovery of the atria are disorganized and chaotic.
- Atrial deflections are irregular.
- Numerous rounded or spiked waves of varying shapes, height and width.

Atrial Flutter

- Expression of rapid and regular atrial excitation
- Presence of regular, undulating, closely spaced, relatively wide atrial deflections/flutter-F-waves in lead II, III, aVF
- Baseline is corrugated—sawtooth appearance

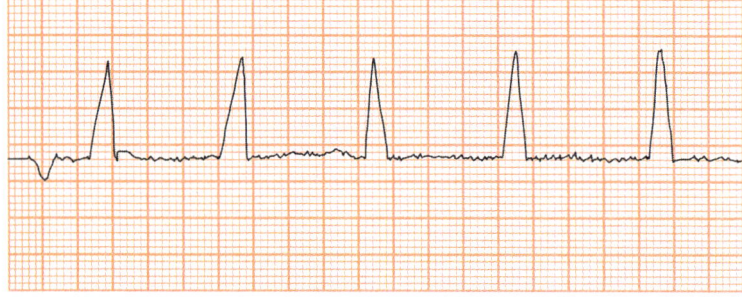

Fig. 15.1: Atrial fibrillation

- Normal QRS complex
- Seen in chronic rheumatic valvular disease, hypertension.

Ventricular Fibrillation

- Expression of chaotic, uncoordinated, ventricular depolarization.
- Numerous rounded or spiked waves of varying shapes, height and width.

Ventricular Flutter

- Uncommon
- Grossly abnormal ventricular conduction
- Rapid regular ectopic ventricular discharge
- QRS and T wave deflections are wide and bizarre.

Supraventricular Tachycardias

- Rapid regular, narrow complex tachycardia
- 220–320 bpm in children
- P wave invisible, or if visible is abnormal in axis
- Retrograde P waves—P wave may precede or follow the QRS.

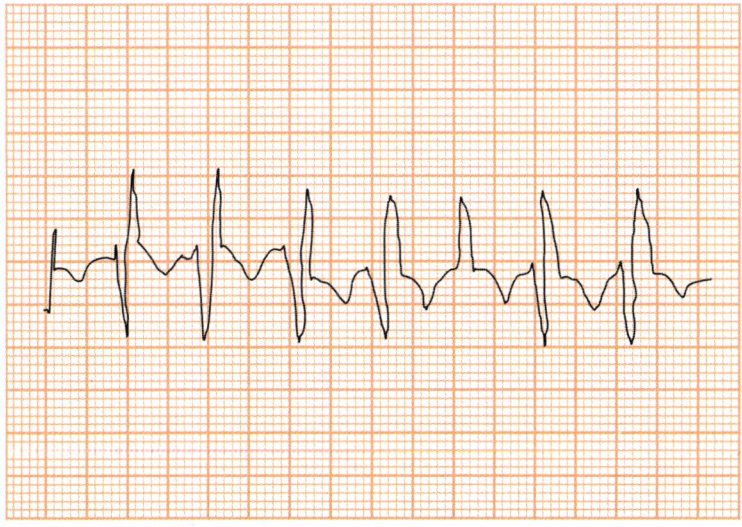

Fig. 15.2: Supraventricular tachycardias

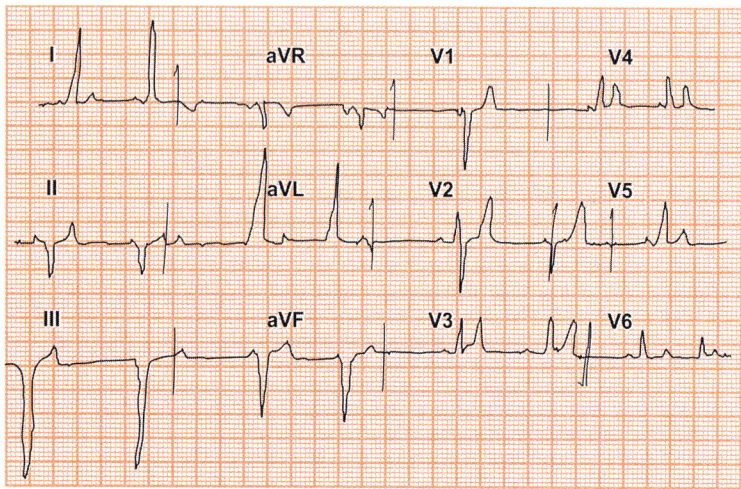

Fig. 15.3: Wolff-Parkinson-White syndrome

Wolff-Parkinson-White Syndrome

- Occurrence of SVT plus specific ECG findings in sinus rhythm.
- Short PR interval and widened QRS with a slurred upstroke or delta wave.
- Caused by earlier ventricular excitation.

16

Miscellaneous

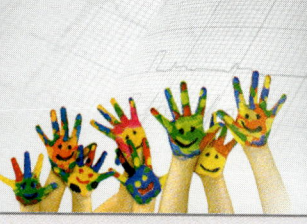

Systemic Hypertension

- Left ventricular hypertrophy due systolic overload
- Long standing case shows left axis deviation
- Earliest and only sign of systemic hypertension is ECG changes of left atrium.
- T wave in lead V1 is taller than V6.
- U wave becomes more inverted in left oriented.
- Left ventricular hypertrophy (LVH) diagnosis by electro-cardiogram (ECG) in hypertensive patients.

Acute Rheumatic Carditis

- Invariable sinus tachycardia
- First degree AV block
- Increased amplitude of upright or inverted T wave
- Depression or elevation of ST segment
- Prolonged QTc interval

Rheumatic Mitral Stenosis

- Left atrial abnormality
- Right QRS axis deviation
- Wide frontal plane QRS-T angle
- Atrial fibrillation
- Wide notched P waves in lead I and V4–6

Digitalis Toxicity

- Characteristic inverse check mark configuration of ST segment
- Tall R wave

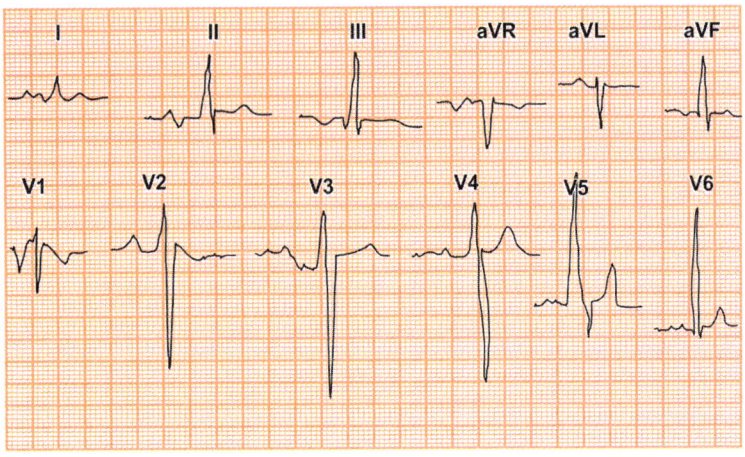

Fig. 16.1: Acute rheumatic carditis

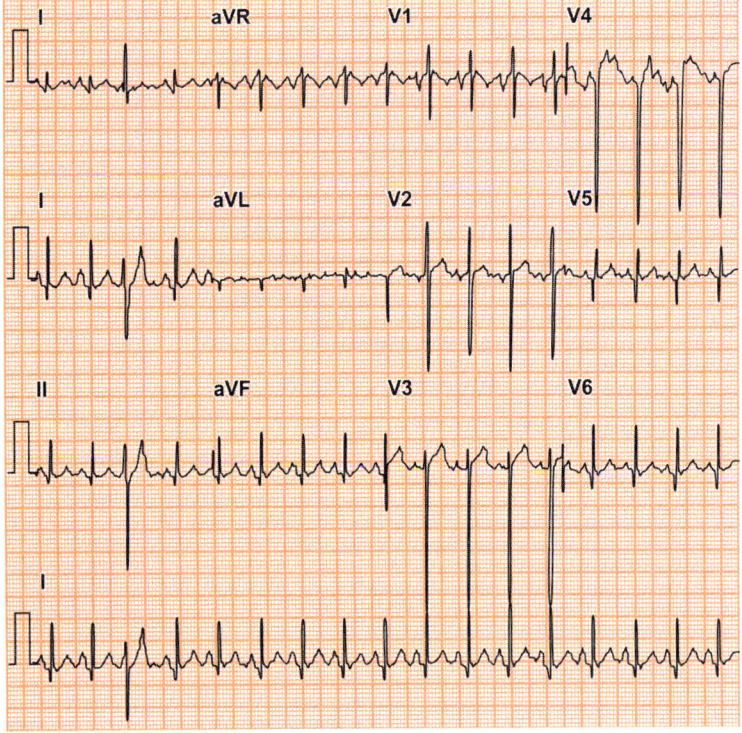

Fig. 16.2: Acute rheumatic carditis ECG

- Shortening of the QT interval
- Paroxysmal atrial tachycardia with block
- Slightly prominent U wave

Mitral Valve Prolapse

- Floppy mitral valve (Barlow syndrome)
- Systolic billowing of one or both mitral leaflets in the left atrium
- Inverted T wave in lead II, III, aVF
- Widened frontal plane QRS-T angle
- T wave inversion in precordial leads
- Sharp angeled ST-T junction
- Prolongation of QT interval
- Atrial and ventricular arrhythmias

Hypothermia

- J waves (also called Osborne waves) are pathognomonic for hypothermia
- Development of J wave at the junction of distal limb of QRS complex with ST segment
- PR segment depression
- Prolongation of QRS complex

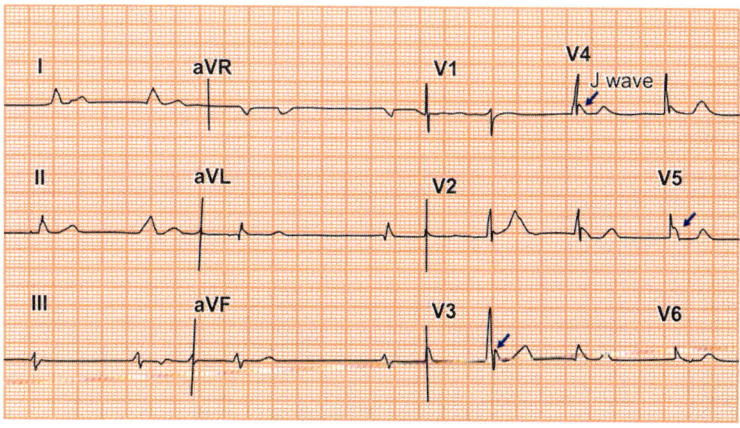

Fig. 16.3: Systemic hypothermia

Table 16.1: Normal values of childhood electrocardiogram

Age	Heart rate	Frontal plane QRS vector (degrees)	PR interval (sec)	QRS duration V5	Q III (mm)	Q V6 (mm)	R V1 (mm)	SV 1 (mm)	R/S V1	RV 6 (mm)	SV (mm)	R/S V6	SV 1+ RV 6 (mm)	R + S V4 (mm)
Less than 1 day	93–154 (123)	+59 to –163 (137)	0.08–0.16 (0.11)	0.03–0.07 (0.05)	4.5	2	5–26 (14)	0–23 (8)	0.1–U (2.2)	0–11 (4)	0–9.5 (3)	0.1–U (2.0)	28	52.5
1 to 2 days	90–159 (123)	+64 to –161 (134)	0.08–0.14 (0.11)	0.03–0.07 (0.05)	6.5	2.5	5–27 (14)	0–21 (9)	0.1–U (2.2)	0–12 (4.5)	0–9.5 (3)	0.1–U (2.5)	29	52
3 to 6 days	91–166 (129)	+77 to –163 (132)	0.07–0.14 (0.11)	0.03–0.14 (0.05)	5.5	3	3–24 (13)	0–17 (7)	0.1–U (2.2)	0.5–12 (5)	0–10 (3.5)	0.1–U (2.2)	24.5	49
1 to 3 wks	107–182 (148)	+65 to +161 (110)	0.07–0.14 (0.10)	0.03–0.08 (0.05)	6	3	3–12 (11)	0–11 (4)	0.1–U (2.2)	2.5–16.5 (7.5)	0–10 (3.5)	0.1–U (3.3)	21	49
1 to 2 mo	121–179 (14)9	+31 to +113 (74)	0.07–0.13 (0.10)	0.03–0.08 (0.05)	7.5	3	3–8 (10)	0–12 (5)	0.1–U (2.2)	5–21.5 (11.5)	0–6.5 (3)	0.2–U (4.8)	29	53.5

(Contd.)

Table 16.1: Normal values of childhood electrocardiogram (Contd.)

Age	Heart rate	Frontal plane QRS vector (degrees)	PR interval (sec)	QRS duration V5	Q III (mm)	Q V6 (mm)	R V1 (mm)	SV 1 (mm)	R/S V1	RV 6 (mm)	SV (mm)	R/S V6	SV 1+ RV 6 (mm)	R + S V4 (mm)
3 to 5 mo	106–186 (141)	+7 to +104 (60)	0.07–0.15 (0.11)	0.03–0.08 (0.05)	6.5	3	3–20 (10)	0–17 (6)	0.1–U (2.2)	6.5–22.5 (13)	0–10 (3)	0.2–U (6.2)	35	61.5
6 to 11 mo	109–169 (134)	+6 to +99 (56)	0.07–0.16 (0.11)	0.03–0.08 (0.05)	8.5	3	1.5–20 (9.5)	0.5–18 (4)	0.1–U (2.2)	6–22.5 (12.5)	0–7 (2)	0.2–U (7.6)	37	53
1 to 2 yr	89–151 (119)	+7 to +101 (55)	0.08–0.15 (0.11)	0.04–0.08 (0.06)	6	3	2.5–17 (9)	0.5–21 (8)	0.1–U (2.2)	6–22.5 (13)	0–6.5 (2)	0.3–U (9.3)	39	49.5
3 to 4 yr	73–137 (108)	+6 to +104 (155)	0.09–0.16 (0.12)	0.04–0.08 (0.06)	5	9.5	1–18 (8)	0.2–21 (10)	0.1–U (2.2)	8–24.5 (15)	0–5 (1.5)	0.6–U (10.8)	42	53.5
5 to 7 yr	65–133 (100)	+11 to +143 (65)	0.09–0.16 (0.12)	0.04–0.08 (0.06)	4	4.5	0.5–14 (4)	0.3–24 (12)	0.1–U (2.2)	8.5–26.5 (16)	0–4 (1)	0.9–U (11.5)	47	54

(Contd.)

Table 16.1: Normal values of childhood electrocardiogram (Contd.)

Age	Heart rate	Frontal plane QRS vector (degrees)	PR interval (sec)	QRS duration V5	Q III (mm)	Q V6 (mm)	R V1 (mm)	SV 1 (mm)	R/S V1	RV 6 (mm)	SV (mm)	R/S V6	SV 1+ RV 6 (mm)	R + S V4 (mm)
8 to 11 yr	62–130 (91)	+9 to +114 (61)	0.08–0.16 (0.11)	0.04–0.09 (0.06)	3	3	0–12 (5.5)	0.3–25 (12)	0.1–U (2.2)	9–25.5 (16)	0–4 (1)	1.5–U (14.3)	45.5	53
12 to 15 yr	60–119 (85)	+11 to –130 (159)	0.08–0.16 (0.11)	0.04–0.09 (0.07)	3	3	0–10 (4)	0.3–21 (11)	0.1–U (2.2)	6.5–23 (14)	0–4 (1)	1.4–U (14.7)	41	50

- Depression of ST segment
- Low to inverted T wave
- Prolongation of QT interval
- Irregular, low amplitude, bizarre oscillations due to shivering
- Sinus bradycardia
- First and second degree AV block
- Ectopic rhythms
- Osborne wave—characterized by a notch in the downward portion of the R wave in the QRS complex.
- Low voltage
- Bradycardia
- Baseline artifact from shivering.

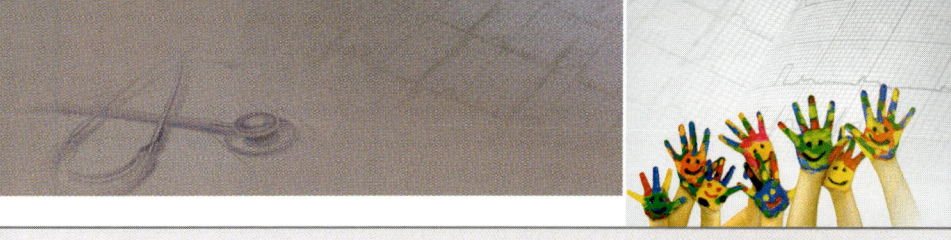

Bibliography

1. Cardiac electrophysiology: Normal and ischemic ionic currents and the ECG Richard E. Klabunde Biomedical Sciences College of Osteopathic Medicine, Marian University, Indianapolis, Indiana, Adv Physiol Educ 41:29–37,2017.

2. Congenital heart disease and the electrocardiogram, MD George Eisenberg , Cardiac Service of Children's Memorial Hospital, Chicago, Ill. USA, The Journal of Pediatrics i Volume 19, Issue 4, Pages 452–469.

3. Guidelines for the interpretation of the neonatal electrocardiogram. A Task Force of the European Society of Cardiology Schwartz PJ (Chair), Garson A, Jr, Paul T, Stramba-Badiale M, European Heart Journal (2002) 23, 1329–1344 doi:10.1053/euhj.2002.3274, available online at http://www.idealibrary.com

4. How to use the 12-lead ECG to predict the site of origin of idiopathic ventricular arrhythmias. Enriquez A, Baranchuk A, Briceno D, Saenz L, Garcia F. Heart Rhythm. 2019 Apr 4.

5. https://en.ecgpedia.org/wiki/Chamber_Hypertrophy_and_Enlargment

6. https://en.wikipedia.org/wiki/Alexander_Muirhead

7. https://en.wikipedia.org/wiki/Augustus_Desir%C3%A9_Waller#cite_note-:0-1

8. https://en.wikipedia.org/wiki/Taro_Takemi

9. https://en.wikipedia.org/wiki/Willem_Einthoven

10. https://www.atlantichealth.org/conditions-treatments/childrens-health/pediatric-cardiology/pediatric-cardiology-diagnostic-tests-screenings/pediatric-electrocardiogram.html

11. https://www.childrenscolorado.org/doctors-and-departments/departments/heart/tests/ekg/

12. https://www.healio.com/cardiology/learn-the-heart/ecg-review/ecg interpretation-tutorial/introduction-to-the-ecg

13. https://www.starship.org.nz/guidelines/ecg-the-neonatal-electrocardiograph/

14. https://www.unboundmedicine.com/harrietlane/view/Harriet_Lane_ Handbook/309501/all/TABLE_7_4:_Normal_Pediatric_ Electrocardio- gram__ECG__Parameters.

15. https://www.utmb.edu/pedi_ed/CoreV2/Cardiology/cardiologyV2/ cardiologyV215.html

16. Normal limits for pediatric electrocardiogram in Ilorin, Nigeria Afolabi Joseph Kolawole, S. I. Omokhodion1 Departments of Paediatrics and Child Health, University of Ilorin Teaching Hospital, Ilorin, 1 Depart- ment of Paediatrics, University College Hospital, Ibadan, Nigeria, Nigerian Journal of Cardiology | July-December 2014 | Vol 11 | Issue 2.

17. paediatric electrocardiography- Steve Goodacre, Karen McLeod BMJ 2002; 324 doi: https://doi.org/10.1136/bmj.324.7350.1382 (Published 08 June 2002)

18. Paediatric electrocardiography-Steve Goodacre and Karen McLeod,, BMJ. 2002 Jun 8; 324(7350): 1382–1385. doi: 10.1136/bmj.324.7350. 1382, PMCID: PMC1123332, ABC of clinical electrocardiography, Electrocardiography, Michael J. Shea.

19. Paediatrics Electrocardiography: Afolabi JK Oloko GYA. Niger J Paed 2012;39 (2):84–89

20. Simplified Pediatric Electrocardiogram Interpretation, William N Evans, MD, Ruben J Acherman, MD, Gary A Mayman. Clinical Pediatrics, Volume: 49 issue: 4, page(s): 363–372.

21. The History Corner: The Galvanometer, Nick Joyce and David Baker.

22. The normal ECG in childhood and adolescence David F Dickinson, Heart. 2005 Dec; 91(12): 1626–1630.doi: 10.1136/hrt.2004.057307.

23. The pediatric electrocardiogram part III: Congenital heart disease and other cardiac syndromes.O'Connor M1, McDaniel N, Brady WJ. Am J Emerg Med. 2008 May;26(4):497–503. doi: 10.1016/j.ajem.2007.08. 004.

24. The pediatric electrocardiogram: part I: Age-related interpretation. O'Connor M1, McDaniel N, Brady WJ. Am J Emerg Med. 2008 May; 26(4):506–12.

25. The pediatric electrocardiogram-Part I: Age-related interpretation, Matthew O'Connor, Nancy McDaniel, William J Brady, American Journal of Emergency MedicineMay 2008Volume 26, Issue 4, Pages 506–512.

26. Dr Lewis Potter. What is Cardiac Axis? https://geekymedics.com/what- is-cardiac-axis/

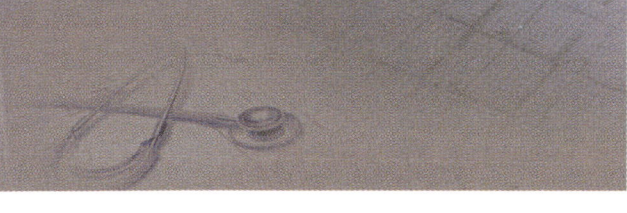
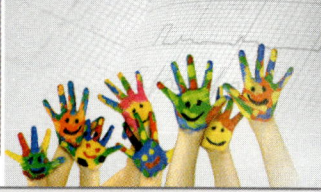

Index